The Fine Art of
UNDERSTANDING
PATIENTS

BY RICHARD C. BATES, M.D.

MEDICAL ECONOMICS BOOK DIVISION, INC.
ORADELL, NEW JERSEY

Second Edition, 1972

CONTENTS

PREFACE

Most practicing doctors would probably jump at a chance to write a discourse such as this on the art of medicine. In time, every practitioner develops a unique style of practice—a philosophy, certain tricks and phrases—that he finds enjoyable and productive. But such is the isolation of private practice that his art is largely hidden from his peers—other doctors—who might be expected to appreciate it most.

What follows is largely a description of *my* art, presented as a "one-man show" for the reader's viewing.

I have no quarrel with people who try to reduce everything in medicine to scientific, reproducible fact—they've accomplished a lot—but the fact remains that a great deal of clinical medicine *is* an art. The science of medicine is concerned with the relationships of health and disease. The art of medicine is directed to the relationships of certain human beings with each other. Like art of any kind, it serves its purpose when the human mind and spirit are uplifted and enriched by it.

Of course, there are risks in publicly pretending to be an artist. As students we could tell which of the old boys was slipping in the science of medicine by the amount of time he devoted to doctor-patient relationships. We called this material by an obscene name and annually awarded a silver shovel to the man who spread it most widely. But we did it with affection, partly because we enjoyed the relaxation of listening to material that wouldn't be included in examinations, but also because these teachers had fleshed out their image as human beings. Still, there was left the impression that the art of medicine and the science of medicine are not complementary but antithetical.

That notion has probably done a lot of harm to patients and to our public image, but it's been very helpful to my pretensions as an expert in the field. Since there are no courses in the art of medical practice—no examinations or "boards"—anyone can hang out his shingle as a specialist.

I can even live with the recognition that my eagerness to accept the challenge of this title means that I've slipped beyond the scientific pale. I used to think that those older professors lost their science because they were too aged or lazy to "keep up." Now I think maybe they had discovered that the best part of being a physician isn't the part in which a man overawes a gaggle of students on rounds by demonstrating his recall of medical minutiae. It's the part, I'm now convinced, in which a doctor is so artful in dealing with people that he can help them feel better even when science can't heal them.

The art of medicine lies in the promotion of productive doctor-patient relationships. Productive relationships are those most efficient in changing sick people for the better. "Efficient" means that one produces the greatest benefit with the least effort in the shortest time. "Art" means that each of us is free to develop his own style, and that some will be naturally gifted while others will succeed only through long and constant practice.

This "show" is presented to affirm that it is possible, in many instances, to enjoy sick, unhappy, difficult people; it *is* possible to charm the cantankerous, motivate the mulish, and please the implacable without pain or loss of self-respect on either side.

In order to promote such productive relationships, one must first thoroughly understand the two parties (or more) who enter into the medical contract. In a contractual agreement, as everyone knows, each party gives up something in exchange for something else. Each party anticipates obtaining "value received," and when he doesn't get it he's apt to be bitter. When a doctor is bitter about a patient or a patient about a doctor, it's usually because the contract went awry.

So we'll start by discussing the parties of the first and second part and their expectations. But the doctor-patient contract seldom succeeds when painted in such drab business hues; it needs to glow with the warmth of a marriage contract. "Doctor," "patient," "productivity," "intimacy," "love": These are the words that appear repeatedly on the pages that follow because they are the primary colors of the art of medicine.

I'm indebted to Erich Fromm, whose writings have taught me about love, and to Eric Berne, whose insights on games throw a spotlight on nonproductive medical practices. Much of what I've learned has been taught me by thousands of dry and drinking alcoholics who demonstrate that intimacy is to cancers of the character what cautery is to cancers of the colon.

The editors of MEDICAL ECONOMICS conceived this book and have been wonderfully helpful in its birth. But best of all for me has been their insistence that it be a one-man show—art can't be produced by a committee.

Richard C. Bates, M.D.
Lansing, Michigan
May 1968

CHAPTER 1

Pinnacles Are
Lonely Places

Since this is to be a book about doctor-patient relationships, let's
begin by taking a look at today's doctor. Obviously, no two
doctors are identical, so that a single portrait of the modern
physician would be as inaccurate as the pictures we are shown of
the wonderful old doctor of yesteryear. But if one had to pick
some adjectives to fit most of the card-carrying practitioners of
today's medicine, he'd certainly include "busy," "harassed,"
"tired." I'd like to add "dissatisfied," "uneasy," "restless," and
"unrequited" to that list.

It seems to me that many of the doctors of today don't achieve
the rewards in medicine that they anticipated at the start. That
brings up the question of what leads young people to choose
medical careers in the first place. It's a key question, because our
fatigue is going to increase until we can attract more help.

The evidence that we're unhappy rests on the facts that our

suicide rate is the highest among all the professions* and that a smaller proportion of our sons go into medicine than was formerly the case. I think the large, recent migration of practicing doctors into salaried work is also an expression of unrest.

Would-be medics are often tested with the question: "Why do you want to be a doctor?" I've never been sure of the proper answer. "To make a lot of money" is the *wrong* one, although at that point in poverty, financial security must loom large on most young men's horizons. The reasons, whatever they may be at the start, probably change during school because medical school changes most of us. Young men tend toward idealism, so maybe some of them are primarily impelled by a genuine desire to relieve suffering humanity. For the weak and inferiority-plagued applicant, there has been (until recently, at least) the attraction of the prestige that goes with being a physician, as well as the promise of opportunities to make godlike decisions and to order people about. Looking back, I think many of my classmates simply identified with a certain doctor—often a father—and wanted to be what he was. Some have said we sought medical secrets in order to postpone our own deaths as long as possible. If there are sexual reasons, they are probably that doctorhood permits asexual promiscuous intimacy—legal voyeurism.

Perhaps curiosity is a large part of it: "I want to get inside people: to find out how they're built, how they run, and how to fix them." If so, there must be an echo: ". . . so I can know more about myself." Then there must be many who eventually find out things about others that they don't want to know about themselves, or who, at least, have all their questions answered. At such a time, a man would either require a new set of reasons for being a doctor or thereafter find medicine dull and unsatisfying.

---

*Psychiatrists, who claim the highest rate of satisfaction with their choice of a specialty, have the highest suicide rate among doctors.

One thing the doctor-in-the-street feels is anger, bewilder-ment, and frustration over the public image of the medical profession. We've been the target of some terribly critical books recently: Roul Tunley's "The American Health Scandal," Ralph L. Smith's "The Health Hucksters," Morton Mintz's "The Thera-peutic Nightmare," William Michelfelder's "It's Cheaper to Die," Richard Carter's "The Doctor Business," an anonymous work titled "The Healers," and Ruth Mulvey Harmer's "American Medical Avarice." And when Parade magazine asked 1,200 adults in 1962, "What do you think of the medical profession today?" nearly one in three declared themselves disappointed in today's doctor.

Still, according to several other surveys, most patients feel their own personal physician is the exception, a "good guy." Other surveys have shown that we are second only to Supreme Court justices in public esteem.

Of course, we don't need to feel lonesome in the stocks of public opinion—other professions also have their critics. Law-yers have been called crooks and big businessmen have been castigated as robber barons who grind the faces of their workers to extract the last penny of profit. Recently, undertakers and automobile and pharmaceutical manufacturers have joined the ranks of the vilified.

Accordingly, it would be easy to rationalize that we are unfair-ly caught in a human need to reduce power figures to the com-mon level. Certainly it is human to condemn certain people collectively (for example, Negroes, Communists, alcoholics) while reserving the right to like those few members of such an out-group that we know as individuals. "Doctors are money-hungry, but my personal physician is a wonderful person" echoes the racist's "Niggers will steal you blind, but our Nellie is just like a member of the family."

We could project the difficulty on the patient and say that he expects too much of us: limitless patience, tact, time, Herculean cheerfulness, gentleness. While we may consider our primary functions to be the retarding of deterioration and death and the alleviation of pain, patients look to us as cardinal sources of reassurance, intimacy, and warmth. Many think of the doctor as the person to whom they would most willingly confide an embarrassing personal secret.

To a scientific, busy practitioner, however, time spent as a father confessor is time wasted, and the prime art of medicine becomes skill in getting people out the door before they start to chat. Our most frequent defense would be identical with our most frequent offense: We're too busy taking care of disease to take care of people. While we would like to enjoy the prestige and gratitude that shower the personal counselor, many of us find that role time-consuming, unscientific, and outside our medical school training. Buffeted by a waiting room full of patients, a woman in labor, and a 12-hour, 40-patient day, we may have to appear brusque to the lonesome old maid whose only other dependable friend is her irritable bowel—even as we recognize that she is hurt and disappointed.

It could be agreed that sick people are often difficult and cantankerous, so that we often get hit by misdirected resentments which should be better aimed at fate, society, personal neglect, or family frictions. Yet we can refute each excuse in turn: Not all professions are attacked by the public. Bankers and stockbrokers, the butts of public ire in the 1930s, now project images of friendliness, sincerity, and helpfulness; teachers and ministers generally escape severe or prolonged criticism.

As for handling difficult people, some doctors get along well with almost everybody, and some of the busiest doctors have the best approach to patients—which is why they're in such demand. And to treat diseases divorced from the people who harbor them is not only difficult but highly inefficient, because our medicine works best in an atmosphere of trust and affection. The remedy for being too busy lies in the direction of becoming more efficient and effective; in medicine this usually means becoming *less* abrupt and impersonal.

We were not always so disliked. Why are we compared unfavorably with bygone doctors? Why did grandfather's doctor meet patients' needs better than we? One reason is that he had more competition. Since the Flexner Report of 1910 eliminated medical diploma mills, we have been in a sellers' market. Before that, many physicians had to supplement their incomes by operating small businesses such as drug and furniture stores because the supply of physicians exceeded the demand. (Dr. Flexner was not solely responsible for this shift, of course—Grandma didn't use the doctor as much as Granddaughter does.)

Physicians of those times are thought of as having been deliberate, patient, kindly, soul-healing individuals—all the things we are now accused of *not* being. But in those days physicians had less work and more free time than they wanted; it was a buyers' market. Now we are in such unhappy short supply that, in some areas, people must beg to be taken on as patients.

Still, I have the uncomfortable feeling that being busier is not the real reason we don't come up to the old doctor in our patients' estimation and that we fail to collect the rewards of being a doctor—rewards that were his in such measure that he was sometimes careless to the point of poverty about collecting his bills.

I think a man's enjoyment of medicine is in direct proportion to his ability to doff the professional mask and enjoy a "people to people" relationship with his patients. If so, the failure of latter-day doctors to achieve such intimacy is at once the prime source of our frustrations and our patients' disappointment.

What are the barriers that hold us back? I suspect some of our difficulty lies in fears of being human. Not only do we fear that our magical, witch-doctor potency will vanish if we take off the professional mask, we share with laymen a universal fear of the risks and responsibilities involved in intimate relationships with others. Doctors are not immune to distrust of strangers or to fear that others may discover our secrets and use that knowledge against us. Doctors can be shy too.

Then there's the fear that our pretense of omnipotence will be shattered, coupled with the rationalization that a patient can feel safe only if he believes his doctor is all-knowing. Lest close association reveal our imperfections, some of our members don an "emperor's cloak" of profundity and preoccupation that discourages any questions about the rationale of treatment or even, in some cases, the diagnosis.

It takes self-approval and self-confidence to approach patients as equals. Yet many of us entered the profession to acquire a status of superiority that would put us safely above the demands of equality. Some people (and there are many such in the professions) can relate only to those to whom they feel superior. Some doctors are comfortable only when they can be erect in the presence of those who are horizontal (which may be the origin of the Freudian couch!); many a professor of medicine stands endlessly towering over patients on rounds when he might better sit down.

Sigmund Freud didn't help matters much, either, by equating love with sex. Until recently we've all been afraid that tenderness was a sign of sexual perversion; if all love is a symptom of sex, then a loving doctor is sick.

So our ability to reap the rewards we seek in being doctors depends in large part upon our personal maturity and self-confidence. Only with these attributes can a doctor be open and at ease with others without worrying about possible damage to his ego or threats to his security. A secure person trusts others as he trusts himself; he is not threatened by change or challenge; he sees people as inherently good, so that he can achieve deep and meaningful relations with others while respecting their right to be unique. And he can give and receive constructive criticism with ease and without anger.

One has to look no farther than our medical organizations (assuming that they accurately reflect the rank-and-file doctor's attitude toward the rest of the world) to see how far we are from the attributes of the secure, authentic person described above, and how deep our insecurity is piled. That insecurity can be productive when it drives a man through medical school; it can be tragic when it persists after school and deprives him of the love and praise he thought would be his reward for all that hard work.

An old doctor I knew as a boy had a framed dictate in his waiting room: "Don't call me 'Doc'; call me 'Doctor'—I worked hard for that title; don't corrupt it." After such an obvious confession that he couldn't tolerate friendliness, it's not surprising that he used to get drunk in the office after evening hours and call his few fishing buddies on the telephone at all hours of the night. Even drunk, he could be friendly only at telephone distance.

Setting oneself up as "Doctor" instead of "Doc" or "Dick" exacts a dreadful price in isolation from mankind; pinnacles are lonely places. Furthermore, it means that one must constantly act the part.

One of the great barriers to productive relationships (and in other fields besides our own) arises from the fallacy of stereotypes. Say "priest" or "labor leader" or "alcoholic" or "doctor," and an image comes to mind of the typical bearer of that label; most people could agree on common attributes for each such type.

Accordingly, a young man coming into medicine tends to believe that he must play the role prescribed by the doctor-stereotype. At this stage he is insecure about his talents, low on the medical totem pole, and conscious of his youth. Protectively, he adopts the plumage of the bird he seeks to be, issuing forth in white coat, stethoscope, reflex hammer, and aloof professional manner. If he *never* grows confident that he is a genuine doctor, he may continue to hide within that plumage for his entire professional career, while relieving the strain of role-playing by hostility toward his patients or family or society, excessive spending, irrational pursuit of sports and hobbies, or addictions.

The more "professional" a person is—the more he seems a typical stereotype of the mass image of his station in life, and the more he insists on looking like (and being treated like) that image—the less likely he is to be a confident, happy, productive person. It is axiomatic that a person who acts a part is pretending to be what he is not. Such a person, then, is clearly dissatisfied with what he thinks he *is*. A physician who is dissatisfied with himself will seldom *be* himself. He can act as he thinks doctors should act and think as doctors are told to think by their leaders, but he will be devoid of individual identity or personality.

Not only does the strain of such role-playing become almost intolerable in time, but patients generally pierce the disguise and instinctively distrust the pretender. Again and again an approving comment about a popular physician will be: "He's not just a good doctor; he's a wonderful human being."

It's too bad that medical students have, in times past, been taught so well what a good doctor should be, when they might better have spent that time learning about other people and discovering that they and these others are basically alike. Fortunately, new teaching methods designed to help students understand and accept themselves and their patients are catching on. The next generation of doctors should be happier.

For those of us taught under the old methods, it's apparent that the foremost barrier to our happiness, our patients' happiness, and our productivity may lie in our fears of being human, our frequent belief that we personally are undeserving pretenders to the exalted title of "doctor," and the teachings of our forebears that a professional aloofness is the physician's proper mien. Deep down, we yearn to love our patients as deeply as they yearn to know and love us.

It's small wonder that the frustration of that love turns to suicide in some of us and to hostility toward the medical profession in some of them.

CHAPTER 2

The Pathology of Patient Dissatisfaction

"The customer is always right" expresses the belief of many successful businessmen that the purchaser must always be left satisfied and with "value received." Maybe this attitude has spoiled a lot of people into thinking that payment of our fees entitles them to write into the doctor-patient contract any terms they wish.

I've met a few patients like that. Usually they're wealthy businessmen who tell me at the start what services they require and indicate that they're willing to pay for them. It's refreshing to encounter such forthright people occasionally, but I wouldn't like a lot of them as patients because they make me feel like a dispensing machine: Put in the nickel and out comes the gum.

Most of my patients don't seem to have a clear notion of what they *do* expect of me—but they know what they *don't* want, and we both know it when they leave unsatisfied.

There have been lots of surveys to document patients' dissatisfactions with present-day medical care: Aloof, impersonal, distracted, uninterested, and money-hungry are only a few of the adjectives we've collected. They sting a little bit because, in part, they're true.

But another part of patient unhappiness, I think, is customer reaction to disappointment over not receiving the goods one came to purchase, coupled with the frustration of not knowing exactly what it was one came to buy.

There are three kinds of office patients: Those who are well and want to stay that way, those who are sick and want to get well, and those who are well but would like to be sick—if they could do so without pain or death. This last group seems to be the largest and most vocal in its criticism of the medical profession, so let's look at them first.

"I went to the doctor for a cold and all he did was give me aspirin and then he charged me five bucks." Sound familiar? I think it's a good springboard from which to dive into the pool of patient expectations. When I hear that comment it tells me that the speaker consulted the doctor because he felt he had a legitimate illness of medical importance. I gather that he expected the doctor to believe so, too. Since most people don't go to doctors for the common cold, I conclude that he must be either stupid, unusually apprehensive about himself, or, more likely, in need of the secondary gains illness provides: an excuse to stop producing, a means of getting concern and sympathy from others, and relief from monotony.

I hear him saying that he expected some dramatic treatment— penicillin or a throat swabbing at the very least—to fortify his hope that the illness merited concern. I have little doubt that he would have been quite plucky in the face of a diagnosis of "walking pneumonia" and might even have accepted hospitalization, although his fortitude would probably stop short of pneumonectomy.

Having his cold treated for what it was and in accord with the very best medical principles left him angry and frustrated, so he carps about the bill. Yet he would cheerfully have paid far more for unnecessary (and possibly dangerous) overtreatment.

How would the paragon of doctorship have treated the cold in the good old days? There'd have been a flossier diagnosis—"catarrh with chest congestion," at least—plus a house call or two and involvement of the rest of the family in the application of hot bricks to the feet, mustard plasters, and careful avoidance of drafts. There might even have been the drama of a "crisis" or a "relapse."

I remember smelling from the street the onion poultices with which our local doctor pulled many people through "incipient pneumonia." And I remember the refined clay with which Mother plastered *my* chest.

Old Doctor would certainly have prescribed several terrible-tasting medicines, compounded and dispensed in his own pharmacy and taken under some peculiar dosage regimen guaranteed to intrigue and involve.* Once when I had a bout of vomiting the doctor came to the house and prescribed a teaspoon of coffee every half hour—for a six-year-old, that's *drama!*

What I'm saying is that scientific knowledge has taken a lot of drama out of people's lives and robbed them of the other gains of illness. I'm *not* saying that old Doc was a charlatan. He really believed in those remedies—it was easy, away from the chilly certitude of double-blind, randomly selected, controlled studies.

So we come to a mutually frustrating impasse. PATIENT: I've got a cold; do me something. DOCTOR: It's a self-limited viral infection; proprietary remedies suffice.

By relieving people of much of the bygone constant fear of death and disease—by doing our job well—we've deprived them

---

*Maybe some of our trouble stems from the pharmaceutical industry's determination to sugar-coat every medicine in sight. Tincture of Iron-Quinine-Strychnine and Syrup of Hydro-iodic Acid: *Those* were remedies a man could believe in!

of some of the savor of life, and I think they dislike us for it. Rousseau expressed some of this in 1762 when he wrote:

"Medicine is all the fashion in these days, and very naturally. It is the amusement of the idle and unemployed, who do not know what to do with their time in taking care of themselves. If by ill-luck they had happened to be immortal, they would have been the most miserable of men; a life they could not lose would be of no value to them. Such men must have doctors to threaten and flatter them, to give them the only pleasure they can enjoy. The pleasure of not being dead."

What's the answer? Certainly not to be charlatans or to encourage people to immoderate indulgence in illness and medical care. Social planners *could* try to put more drama back into people's lives: something short of race riots and far better than current television fare. In time, I expect, the public will adjust to the new warranty of 70 years of life and meet their needs in other ways. In any event, there probably isn't much the doctor-in-the-street can do to promote such mass change.

In the meantime it would help if we could devote more time to the patient who is disappointed and frustrated by the scientific approach to his ills. Not only do we possess more potent scientific nostrums than Grand-doc had for Grandpa, but we also have better psychological insights that could help these people with their *real* problems.

Grand-doc had only first-degree therapy: helping people to get the diagnosis they wanted. We have second-degree therapy which allows us to meet that need with more acceptable substitutes. If a patient gives evidence of wanting drama and attention and concern, why can't that be regarded as a deficiency disease amenable to supplementary feedings with enriched and fortified Tender Loving Care? Only in rare instances would such treatment have to be carried out by the doctor: Generally all he has to do is help the patient be more lovable and arrange for others to dispense the T.L.C. (Best of all is third-degree therapy: helping the patient mature into the sort of person who gives attention and concern to others instead of hungering for it for himself. Usually that requires group therapy.)

Patients who are genuinely sick expect many additional things from us: our concern; undivided time; thoroughness; maturity; wisdom; cleanliness; a modern, well-equipped office; competent and efficient staff members. Near the top of their list, right after T.L.C., I'd place credibility. When a man's only worried about the *possibility* of being sick, our time and concern are adequate remedies, but when there really is a genuine, dangerous illness, I think he'd trade all the T.L.C. in the world for a doctor who could pull him through. With luck, he'll find both, of course.

How does a doctor make himself credible—what are the ingredients for instilling faith? Nothing succeeds like success, so I guess speedy relief of distress would rank high. Certainly a doctor's reputation around town is a valuable therapeutic agent. Personal appearance and an assured manner contribute to a good first impression, and a retinue of eager students is wonderful, if it can be arranged.

But I think frankness and honesty outrank all those. If I were really sick, a doctor who was evasive, ill at ease, and vacillating is the one that would scare me the most. When patients complain that their doctor doesn't spend enough time with them, I think they're often saying that he doesn't communicate enough to let them tell whether he knows his business. So they suspect the worst.

The credibility gap is widest when there is a wide age difference between doctor and patient; it is narrowed by longer acquaintance. It is wider when the doctor is in solo practice, and grows with the distance he practices from a big city. The more education a patient has and the more money he earns, the more suspicious he becomes. The solo practitioner in a small hospital in a small town who's faced with treating the wife of the bank president might as well send her right to the Big Medical Center. Does intimacy narrow the gap? Not if familiarity breeds contempt. A friendly manner certainly suggests that one has nothing to hide, but many people (particularly in lower socio-economic groups and when faced with surgery) figure that a man who's rough and gruff *has* to be good. That illusion is a fortunate one for doctors who are afraid of their patients; sometimes I think it's the only thing that keeps a few of my colleagues in business.

Instead of using gruffness to build confidence, I prefer kindly candor. If I don't know, I say so; if I do know, I don't mince words. Given a patient with sore joints, I say, with a sympathetic smile: "There are several possibilities, including rheumatoid arthritis. We'll run the tests to narrow those possibilities down. We may have to wait and let your disease get bad enough so that we can tell what it is. In any event, I'll let you know as soon as *I* find out. Even though you're uncomfortable, I'd rather not start treatment until we have the diagnosis. Do you have any questions?" This form of presentation is reassuring to *some* people, in any event. The other day a woman called about her mentally deficient child. The authorities were suggesting special schooling, and she didn't trust them. "We've moved across town and go to another doctor now," she began, "but I just had to call you—you were always so frank and honest with us that I know I'll be able to trust *your* advice."

All in all, patients want doctors they can believe in, doctors who are available, doctors who are helpful and satisfying. Eventually, most of them sort themselves out and find the kind of man they want. As noted earlier, most people apparently believe that their personal doctor is a jewel, but that the medical profession as a whole could stand a lot of improving. Maybe they get that attitude from us: I daresay almost every practicing doctor has the same attitude toward himself and his colleagues.

CHAPTER 3

Breaking the
Doctor-Patient Barrier

The word "rapport" is flung at medical students as something they have to have with a patient in order to extract a good history from him. The general impression *I* received, at least, was that I should approach a new patient with an outwardly neutral attitude because, if I showed how I really felt about being assigned another work-up, the subject might retaliate with monosyllabic answers. However, I was always to keep my guard up with a professional bedside manner.

It's small wonder that I never attained, in school, internship, or residency, the kind of rapport that I now regard as the 100-proof, genuine article. As a freshman in school I could have done it, but freshmen weren't exposed to patients, probably because we hadn't yet been taught to be professional.

It's been noted many times that great changes occur between the first and last years of medical school, resulting in the conversion of an eager, loving freshman into a hard, aloof, skeptical, rejecting senior. A lot of verbal head-scratching has taken place over the nature and causes of these changes, because they appear to be common to all medical students. A progressive hostility toward patients arises, reaches its zenith at residency, and (hopefully) declines thereafter.

Though the budding medico is often unaware of his hostility, it's quite obvious to the patient, ward personnel, and older doctors. It shows in frowns, angry tones of voice, gestures, phrases like "gork" and "crock," lack of feeling for patients' privacy or sensitivity, and a preference for thinking of people as cases or diseases rather than as feeling, worrying fellow humans. To the extent that the medical fledgling thinks of "patients" as being different from "friends," he keeps them at stethoscope distance.

When this hostility persists into later practice it hampers a doctor's effectiveness, breeds antagonism toward the whole profession, and, worst of all for him, robs him of the very satisfactions he sought by going into medicine. Fortunately, most of us gradually get over it—looking back, it took me at least 10 years to make the trip.

Where is this hostile attitude spawned? Medical school teachers have been accused of milting it; certainly warmth is less intense among the permanent inhabitants of large medical centers than it is in the boondocks, where a doctor's income may be proportionate to his friendliness. Some teachers of psychiatry, at least, give students a rationalization for aloofness with their injunctions against emotional entanglements and their portrayals of love as a symptom of sex.

A psychologist-friend of mine assures me, however, that the same hostility appears in budding clinical psychologists and social workers. This suggests that it may be common to every student preparing to assume responsibility for helping and healing. If so, the psychiatrists and other professors are partly off the hook. They'll be completely off when they follow the example of a few psychiatry departments such as that at the University of Oklahoma and carry out group therapy to confront the students with their untoward reactions.*

A reaction so universal couldn't be the result of malignant teaching. In order to occur everywhere it must arise as the natural result of some universal forces operating on medical students —and I have a hunch I know what some of those forces are.

Hostility is a nasty, but psychologically appropriate, reaction to threats against the ego. From that point, it's a short hop to the surmise that a student raised to an eminence from which he is expected to heal the sick is assailed by acrophobic insecurity, and that his hostility is a defense against having his insecurity unmasked. If so, we can state that one of the principal requirements for the establishment of rapport is a self-confident doctor.

(Not merely students, but the medical profession as a whole appears to express this fright. When one takes a long view of the ultraconservative reactions of organized medicine, the fascination of many doctors with the acquisition of money or political power, and the defensiveness of our positions against osteopaths, chiropractors, and social planners, it's apparent that the prototype of the American doctor is a man at bay, scared to death that he'll fall or be pushed off the eminence he's scaled.)

It's easy to see why a sophomore medical student on first approach to the bedside feels insecure, particularly if he's introduced falsely to the patient as a doctor. Small wonder he dons a protective cloak of chill impersonality to keep the patient from penetrating his disguise—not that the patient can't tell instantly. I remember *our* first experiences in history-taking. The results were pretty bad except for one of our number who got a very good story from *his* patient—so good that we accused him of having had extern experience. "Not so," he explained. "I told the

---

*See "Some 'Teachable' Aspects of Interviewing," Chester M. Pierce, J. Oklahoma Med. Assn., December 1963.

patient this was my first history and asked him to help me, and he did." The other patients, as I later discovered, knew full well that we were neophytes and made things tough because we were pretending to be something we were not.

Fear of being unmasked as a student is soon over, yet the typical doctor still suffers his hostility-breeding insecurity. The larger fear, I suspect, stems from the risks of intimacy: The hazards of forming close bonds with patients probably stem from the dangers inherent in our side of the contract. Scientists may comfortably look at people as though they were bugs on pins, but therapeutic rapport requires a measure of equality—meaning that the patient can stare back. Let's put it this way: The main deterrent that keeps most people from walking through nudist camps is the rule that visitors must strip, too.

The analogy of the nudist camp is excellent for understanding rapport. I've never been in one, but reporters say that all awkwardness disappears in the first hour and is replaced with a wonderful sense of equality and freedom. The reason is that, without clothes, each camper is divested of pretense and loses the need to maintain or achieve status. The physical examination itself, wherein one gives up all his protective plumage and permits another to examine all accessible areas of his body, is one of our best tools for promotion of rapport. I've noted that one of the results of the examinations I've undergone is a feeling of warmth and affection for my examiner. Perhaps the most important (but largely subconscious) benefit of the yearly physical "game" is this opportunity to expose oneself completely to another. If so, the doctor who never gets his patients' clothes off seldom gets close to the seat of their problems.

But having given his innermost mental and physical secrets to us, the patient requires the reassurance of some intimacy in return. Indeed, we are usually in the position of having to take the first step. My classmate who admitted to his patient that he was a greenhorn thereby took off his own protective plumage first.

That's the main risk of intimacy: It requires something from us, if only that we "put out" to another person in order to penetrate his defenses.

But too many of us in the early days of training are not geared to giving. We go into medicine, in part, to achieve superior status: Gods don't make sacrifices to men. Confronting a patient, we say in effect: "You are so weak that you have to come to me for help. That puts you in my power. If I have power over you, I shouldn't have to give you anything—it ought to be the other way around. Don't come back unless you're prepared to follow orders." In a young student this attitude can be aggravated by the residuals of childhood yearnings to achieve the power over others that his parents have had over him.

Lesser barriers to rapport come from jealousy: "How come this guy gets to go out and get drunk when I have to work for a living?" "Here you are whining about being on a strict bed confinement when I'd give anything to spend all day in bed with pretty nurses to rub my back." Other fears feed fear of intimacy: "If I become personally close to this patient anything dire that afflicts him will pain me." "If I show this woman love she may equate it with sex."

In addition, in comparing my feelings for strong, healthy people and for diseased, sick, weak people, I've identified in myself a distaste for the latter. I don't like disease, and I don't like to see it in people: That's inherent in being a doctor. A fireman hates fire, and a policeman hates crime, and a house painter hates dry rot.

This comes close to a common hang-up in the rapport campaign: the "Why can't people be more like me?" barrier. In medicine it takes such forms as, "Anybody can quit smoking (drinking, overeating)—I did"; "Poor people are too lazy to work hard for a living as I do"; and "You'd be in good health if you'd take care of yourself." A doctor, then, may tend to see himself as healthy (good) (strong) (wholesome) and feel that most of the sick are self-indulgent weaklings who deserve no sympathy.

Applied to day-to-day practice, all this boils down to an attitude I repeatedly guard myself against. It goes like this: "This patient is going to try to keep me from penetrating to the core of his personality because, while he'd very much like such a relationship, he's afraid of nakedness. I'm afraid of him, too, because he jeopardizes my image as an all-knowing god rather than a mere man—a Wizard of Oz, mainly humbug. If I show emotion, it will indicate that I'm human and then he'll lose respect for me. He may even dominate me and will certainly require equal, if not superior, status. This will mean that I have to 'put out' as much as I take in, or even give *more* than I get."

So much for the antithesis of rapport: What of the thesis? I suppose every individual has his own secret ways of winning friends and influencing people. Briefly, I think the ingredients include:

Respect—for a patient's rights to privacy, freedom of choice, the right to be different.

Tolerance—for human weakness.

Knowledge—of oneself and of the wide spectrum of human behavior.

Generosity—willingness to give more than one gets.

Honesty—to be frank and natural and to admit frailty and fallibility.

Trust, faith—that people are inherently good, no matter how ornery they appear.

Confidence—that others will not take advantage of intimacy; that one can control oneself and tolerate the risks of a two-way contract.

Care—about and for others. Care for strong things, weak

things, crippled and straight—"reverence for life," Schweitzer called it.

Discipline—willingness to be firm in setting others on the path toward becoming lovable, as well as self-discipline to continue one's own growth and improvement.

It's common in a treatise like this to go into the differences between empathy and sympathy and to repeat the medical shibboleth that empathy is fine but sympathy is bad. I don't believe it, and the frequency with which professionals bring the topic up makes me suspect they're only excusing their own fears of personal involvement. The more I practice, the more sympathy I feel—and show. My experience is that an ounce of sympathy is worth a pound of empathy, if anyone can really separate the two. When I feel sorry for a patient I feel equal to him. When I tell him I feel sorry for him, it's a lot more productive than the old empathy bit that says "I know how you feel and that it's unpleasant, but I must hold myself apart from your suffering." When my patients get tears in their eyes and I'm on the right rapport wavelength, I get tears too and take the risk of admitting it: "I notice your eyes are moist and I'll have to confess that seeing you so sad makes me sad too. What can I do to help?" Being able to give genuine sympathy is not a sign of weakness but of strength; empathy is neutral, sympathy is positive. To me, sympathy equals empathy plus personal involvement.

Sometimes rapport is almost instantaneous. A new patient comes in; he appears to be my sort of person; I flash him a smile, and he flashes one back: In that moment each of us has said, "I like you."

At other times rapport has to be earned laboriously. Some people have been hurt so many times when they've risked intimacy that they're as skittish as a little wild squirrel: Every time I take a slow step forward, they run back two. But they're the ones who most need the proffered nut.

Generally, the nearer a patient is to my age the easier it is to harmonize, but that doesn't mean one has to act like a kid to get along with adolescents or like an old goat to approach the aged.

With youngsters I often get good results with gay, direct confrontation: "Hey, you look scared to death!" or "Something tells me you don't like doctors much" or "Cheer up, I've never lost a patient during a physical exam yet." What's said isn't nearly as important as how it's said, and a grin is the most effective weapon in my arsenal.

With luck, I convey in this first greeting the messages "I like teenagers; I know how you feel; I don't blame you for being ill at ease; I'll help you through this; I'm not at all like the stern, awesome, authority figure you expected—let's make this fun."

With oldsters my approach is less aggressive, more mature, loving, and sympathetic. Usually older people have lost most of their childhood fear of doctors, but they've accreted layers of protective reserve against strangers. Having passed the zenith, they often feel inferior—"used up" or a "has been"—so they usually want to impress me with what they once were. Men boast about their life's work, women about their descendants. So I bring these subjects up as soon as it can gracefully be done. No matter how meagre their accomplishments, I can be admiring so long as I forget myself and become immersed in them. This ability to forget oneself in order to become totally merged in another is a high skill, wonderfully conducive to rapport.

In addition to training myself to smile as much as possible, I've had to learn to *touch people* and to *use first names*. These hallmarks of intimacy must usually be initiated by the doctor, at the risk of having the patient reciprocate. Many of us were taught, I think wrongly, to avoid both of them.

When a new patient arrives, I shake his hand warmly; in the hospital, I always pat a hand or the patient's arm as I step up to the bed; after a "tough" and tearful psychiatric interview I put an arm around a patient's shoulders as he leaves. Never have I had a patient take these gestures amiss.

When a patient between the ages of 30 and 70 persistently "sirs" or "doctors" me, I confront him with: "You know, when you call me 'sir' it makes me feel as though you were setting me up as your superior officer. Even though I know you are doing it as a mark of respect, the effect is to keep me at arm's length. Suppose you call me "Dick" for a trial and see what happens?" Then I call him "Fred" and marvel at how such a simple thing sweeps away the barriers between us.*

Rapport is not hurried; it is not strained; it is neither forced nor unnatural. Webster defines it as a relationship characterized by harmony, conformity, accord, and affinity; I think of it as an atmosphere that permits productive intimacy. Whatever it is, it's sweet and valuable, artful and lovely. When I'm en rapport with a patient we both know it, we both enjoy it, and we both want it to go on. Almost always, it does.

---

*An exception must be made in the case of Negroes. Despite their desire for equality, Negroes regard being called by their first names as a mark of disrespect, so it's important, at least in the early stages of an association to use "mister" or other appropriate titles.

CHAPTER 4

Your Office Tells
People About You

It's too bad that the people who teach medicine have so little contact with office practice, because his office is where a doctor in private practice spends most of his time. As a result of this professorial inexperience, young doctors are often entirely untrained in the art they most need to get off to a productive start: the art of creating a proper office atmosphere.

The professor of medicine at the university may not need a cheerful, motherly secretary or clean, comfortable furniture to impress his patients and instill reassuring faith. His obvious self-assurance, gray hair, and title should be more than adequate for the task.

But the doctor without medical school prestige—and especially the solo doctor without even group or clinic prestige—must be careful about what his office does to his patients, particularly in the early years of practice before his reputation and competency are established in the community.

Sure, it would be fine if we were judged solely on our medical merits. Maybe we'd like to believe that people stupid enough to choose doctors solely by the thickness of their carpets deserve the kind of care they get. But doctors *are* judged by the decor they keep, and by the help they hire. Nor are these judgments irrational. An office can tell sensitive people—particularly women who pay a great deal of attention to housekeeping and furnishings—a great deal about the inhabitants thereof.

It's not that a doctor wants to dazzle patients with fine feathers in lieu of being a fine bird, nor that first impressions can't be overcome. I certainly wouldn't want to care for people so superficial that they chose me solely on the basis of my color scheme. What's important is that an office can help to create a productive atmosphere of intimacy and relaxation.

An office may indicate how much or little a doctor cares about his patients. What would you be thinking about a man you'd never met while sitting in his office on a cheap plastic chair with broken springs and a cigarette burn in the arm rest? How would you feel about a man whose waiting room reading material consisted wholly of religious tracts?

If an office can express warmth, it can also be cold; if it can be cheerful, it can also be cheerless; if it can be welcoming, it can also express hostility.

How can an office reveal that its owner is hostile to patients? It's easy. First, there's the voice on the telephone when the appointment is made, but that's a chapter all by itself. Then there's the location. A pediatrician's office in a downtown bank building with all the society doctors tells mothers something as they circle the block for the tenth time looking for a parking place.

Seedy, rundown buildings are often inhabited by seedy, rundown businesses run by seedy, rundown businessmen, so our new man in town will be wise to take the added risk of a more expensive suite in a newer building. Chances are the parking space there will be more adequate, too.

The location of the office in the building, the brightness of the corridors, the very lettering on his door will contribute to the image people form of him and of his medicine.

The door opens. Immediately the eye searches for the answer to the number-one question at that moment. It's not whether the secretary is cute, or whether the draperies are bright—it's the question a man has first in mind when he enters a barbershop: How many are waiting ahead of me? Even if no one is waiting at the moment, the presence of a large number of empty chairs may suggest that many people *do* wait there at times, so I'd recommend very few chairs—that's one of the few places where our neophyte can safely economize.

Naturally, the doctor's aides can be an asset or a detriment to patient relationships. If that medical professor's secretary is frosty, everybody will (rightly) assume that she's a relative of the administration or under civil service. But in a private doctor's office they'll assume that the secretary is reflecting her boss's attitude toward people, because he personally hired and trained her.

It's generally considered bad policy for a doctor's wife to work for him, but I'm not sure this is *always* true. In any event, if she does, patients should all be aware of the fact so they won't embarrass themselves by saying things to her as a secretary that they wouldn't say to his wife. And she can expect some curtailment of the number of her personal friends who come to her husband for care.

A warm aide can do a lot to thaw a frosty patient by friendly small-talk or helpful information. Like the doctor, she must be unhurried to do her best. I like to have a name plate for her desk so patients can get to know her as a person as soon as possible. When I hear patients calling my receptionist by her first name I know they're old established friends of both of us. And think how reassuring it must be to the frightened mother of a sick child to hear, at the other end of the telephone line, the friendly voice of a receptionist she knows by name!

If you don't believe that offices can influence patient relationships, listen to some of the comments gathered by a G.P. who secreted a tape recorder in his waiting room:

"Such screaming! Whatever can he be doing to that child?"

"Well, I'm certainly going to close the door when I go in there. From here, you can hear every word the mother is saying."

"The dirt on those walls should deaden any sound! And look at the dust on this table! What kind of cleaning woman has he got, anyway?"

"I wouldn't mind waiting if he'd only put a decent light in here."

Bad lighting is easily fixed, but an office that isn't sound-proof is almost hopeless. Before the new man signs a lease it's essential that he stand in the waiting room and listen while his wife talks in a loud voice in all the back rooms. If he can understand her, he can be pretty sure very few people are going to bare the intimacies of their lives to him in *that* office. If the lease is already signed, some piped-in music for the waiting room may scramble conversations enough to make them unintelligible, but it will have to be kept soft or his front-office help will get scrambled from listening to it.

Ready for some more patient gripes? Here are a few from a survey MEDICAL ECONOMICS reported in its issue of April 20, 1964. The question: "What are a few things you like (or don't like) about your doctor's office?" These were the most frequent retorts:

1. Uncomfortably crowded waiting rooms.

2. Dingy or gloomy offices.

3. Large or lavish offices.

What do they like? Patient after patient praised his doctor's office as being "homey," but the best reactions of all were for newness: "Brand-new office—no complaints" . . . "new—wonderful" . . . "new, modern, comfortable, not one thing wrong with it."

People feel more secure in their homes than in an office. Secure people are likely to open up and talk, so the more an office looks like home and the less like an office, the more productive your interviews are apt to be.

To make an office homey, I'd recommend carpeting throughout, stuffed furniture upholstered with cloth (not plastic), healthy green plants (*certainly* not plastic), and something to express the doctor's personality—to show that he's human. If he has a suitable hobby it might be worked into his decor. (This must be done with discretion, however—I'd wonder about a doctor who had golfing memorabilia all over the place.) At least *some* attempt should be made to make it a little different from any other office in the world, if only to provide a starter for conversation with that friendly receptionist. Tropical fish are great for kids provided somebody cleans the tank once in a millenium.

I like to grow house plants, so in my office you'll find them even in the examining rooms. I like to think that patients judge my skill in caring for people by the number of new shoots I can encourage to sprout above the pots. (That's easily arranged because, unlike patients, sickly plants can be thrown out the back door.)

Now for the history-taking. Volumes could be written on this most sensitive and artful maneuver in medicine—indeed, they have been. A productive person-to-person exchange requires relaxation, intimacy, empathy and compassion, knowledge, mutual respect, and caring. These are the ingredients of Fromm's mature love,° so we might as well break down and say that the

---

°Erich Fromm, "*The Art of Loving,*" Harper & Row, 1956.

history must be taken in a loving fashion—let the pseudo-Freudians snicker as they will. It doesn't mean that the patient sits on the doctor's lap, but it doesn't mean either that he's stretched naked on a paper sheet staring at the ceiling or perched on the edge of a hard table in his underwear. We're usually clothed when conversing with friends, so clothed the patient should be. Nor do we visit with our friends while barricaded behind a desk, so it's best to have the desk (with all its distracting plastic pharmaceutical bric-a-brac) behind the doctor. We use clipboards to take histories in the hospital, so one can be used in the office, or perhaps a chair with an arm board or a desk that stands beside the doctor will do. A low coffee table with an ashtray and a box of tissues for the tearful will suffice to represent the distance that the doctor and patient must be separated. If it contains hot coffee as well, the history will be correspondingly enhanced. Provided that the doctor doesn't become intoxicated with caffeine, it's extraordinary what the ceremony of pouring and sharing coffee can do to break down reticence. Some of the flossier society types are rumored to offer patients cocktails, but in that case I'd recommend that the doctor stick to the coffee and leave the drinking to them.

Dr. Hilton S. Read, a Ventnor, N.J., internist, interviews patients beside a crackling fireplace—at least in the wintertime—which is about as homey as you can get unless you add a rocking chair and a purring cat. I have no doubt that it's a wonderful adjunct to atmosphere (if the chimney draws well). And he and I both eschew the white coat because it's a symbol of "clinical" medicine.

If relaxation is important to a good history, it's *essential* to an accurate physical exam.

The examining room must necessarily be clinical, although a picture or a plant can be squeezed in. I don't like paper sheets or towels—cloth seems much more homey to me, and after all it's the patient who's paying for it. The room should be warm in temperature, but it must be cool in color (I like a soft gray) if skin tones are to come through accurately. I don't know exactly why examining tables have to be hard, narrow, and high, but that seems to be the only way they're made. The room itself may be quite small (if well ventilated), because nakedness seems to be accentuated by big, high-ceilinged rooms. Personally, I don't like to examine people in the presence of a heap of underwear, so I have a screened dressing alcove with coat hooks (desirable) and a mirror (essential). Unless they've had access to a mirror as they dressed, women are too preoccupied with frets about their appearance to hear our final advice and parting shots.

While the patient is dressing, his routine laboratory, height, weight, temperature, and blood pressure data can be collected in preparation for the report. In an efficient office and for a healthy patient, all those materials can be ready in 30 minutes or less.

Ready availability of laboratory services can do a lot to promote efficiency and prevent anxiety. Dr. A sees his patients, looks mysterious, orders some tests at a laboratory across town and some X-rays on another day at the hospital five miles in another direction, and makes an appointment to see the patient again in three weeks for "reports." By then, he's forgotten what it was he was checking for, but his patient isn't apt to forget those sleepless nights of wondering if he has cancer.

Dr. B, in a clinic or medical office building, gets laboratory and X-ray studies in his building on the day he orders them and often gives his patients their reports before they leave.

Normal reports of routine exams that take longer (chest X-rays, Pap smears) can be telephoned by the secretary. But *abnormal* reports should be phoned by the doctor himself so that reassurance can be given and questions answered, while reports of a serious nature should be given face-to-face. For example, it would be most unwise to telephone an unmarried girl the report of a positive pregnancy test. Instead, I try to have her boyfriend or her parents come in with her. If routine reports are handled by telephone, some fail-safe system should be devised to ensure that the call gets made. Such a system is a must for abnormal reports. A doctor can be sued if his secretary mistakenly files a questionable X-ray report that merits further investigation. And it's important to be sure that the word gets to the proper person. I wouldn't suggest trusting a teen-age daughter with the news that her mother should have a repeat Pap smear in three months.

Which brings up the matter of "tickle" files. Many doctors are insecure about their ability to attract and hold patients. They like to feel needed, and they need constant reassurance that everyone they see is genuinely enthusiastic about them. So, to them, it's comforting to place the responsibility for the next appointment on the patient's shoulders. When *he* initiates the contact it shows that he needs and appreciates help.

Patients don't understand this very well, so when a doctor says, "Call me for an appointment in a few weeks," they may feel they're being rejected or at least treated pretty casually. When we meet a friend on the street and part with, "Come and see us sometime," it's a lot cooler relationship than we'd express by saying, "Can you and your wife come for dinner next Thursday evening at 6?"

Furthermore, some patients are careless about making appointments; some repress the memory of our advice because they find any exposure to the medical profession unsettling. And, unlike us, most people don't keep appointment books to which they refer daily.

Therefore, when I want a patient to come back within three months, we give him an appointment as he leaves. For longer waits we make a note in our tickler file—really a second appointment book—to call the patient a few weeks before he's due to return and arrange the appointment then, because the farther an appointment is set ahead the more chance there is that it will be forgotten. From the doctor's standpoint, forgotten appointments are worse than inefficient; they can also be so embarrassing to a sensitive patient that he may never be comfortable in that office again.

Occasionally we have a patient who repeatedly forgets appointments, and for him we have a reminder system. To avoid any implication that we don't trust him, we tell him at the time his appointment is made that "because you're so busy" we'll provide a no-charge extra service by phoning him a reminder on the morning of his appointment date.

For some reason, there's a common but erroneous belief that it's unethical for a doctor to remind patients when it's time for a yearly physical exam. Dentists do it regularly, and their patients appreciate the service. Some doctors instruct their secretaries to ask patients if they'd like to be reminded to return in a year, but for years I've routinely sent a form letter, personally signed, one year after every examination of this sort. To date, no patient has complained. But I did recently hear a bitter complaint from a man whose doctor had discontinued a similar service to his patients without warning them. When this individual discovered that he hadn't had an exam for two years he decided that his doctor was too busy to care about him anymore, and changed doctors.

If a patient wanted to break off it might be embarrassing for him to say so on a personal call from the doctor's secretary, so we send the following printed letter, personally signed.

Dear_____,

According to our records, it has been a year since your last complete examination.

If you wish to make this a yearly habit, please call us for an appointment.

Sincerely yours,

Note that the phrase, "If you wish to make this a yearly habit" clearly indicates that there will be no hard feelings if he doesn't elect to avail himself of this expensive semiluxury.

To sum up, a doctor's office should be available, comfortable, personal, and homey. His routines should preserve privacy, promote tranquillity and efficiency, and "reach out" to people.

CHAPTER 5

The Special Needs of Hospital Patients

The day may not be distant when one set of doctors works entirely on hospitalized patients and another on outpatients. When that day arrives, I'm willing to bet, the doctors who choose bedside care will be those who are more comfortable with guinea pigs than with people, with science than with art, and with facts than philosophies.

Until that time many of us plant a sole in each camp. And that's good, because if anyone needs massive infusions of the art of medicine, heaven knows it's the patient sick enough to be hospitalized.

Yet I have the distinct notion that even those of us who practice both kinds of medicine do a poorer job of caring for the emotional needs of the bedridden than we do of the ambulatory; our deskside manners are more artful than our bedside manners.

Maybe the power we assume in the hospital setting corrupts us. Maybe in the hospital our preoccupation with physical derangements blinds us to the emotional. It could be that we pattern our "professional" hospital mien after those scientists who taught us at the bedside, but have subsequently gone on to develop our own more intimate outpatient techniques in the isolation of our offices.

Privacy is certainly part of the problem, because the majority of hospitalized patients don't have a moment of it from admission to discharge. In particular, they seldom get a moment alone with their doctor. What doctor would take a patient's history in his office waiting room, with other patients listening in? And yet, isn't this precisely the arrangement when one "works up" a hospital patient in a ward bed during visiting hours? How many of us would repeat one patient's case history to the next patient on the office schedule? Yet we think nothing of discussing a hospital patient's case with students while the roommates listen in. I suppose this medieval disregard of personal feelings will continue until someone gets Belli-full of law suits for invasion of privacy. Meanwhile, I wonder if we *ever* get an accurate and intimate history at the bedside.

Not that an entourage is *always* an encumbrance. Patients can't help but be impressed when swarms of students hang on their doctor's every flick of the stethoscope. This awe can be utilized to close the credibility gap or to discipline an unruly patient.

For the first purpose, the doctor simply tells the students something he wants the patient to believe. "I'm happy to report that all of Mr. Smith's X-rays are negative for cancer" when said to students carries twice the assurance of the same message given privately.

As an example of the second purpose, one lectures to students on the evils of smoking at the bedside of an emphysema patient, letting him squirm under ten pairs of disapproving eyes.

But these are the exceptions and come under "treatment."

When it comes to diagnosis, there's no substitute for privacy. Few patients can bring themselves to make intimate revelations in a crowd. I'm inhibited, too, when I try to establish an intimate relationship in the presence of two roommates, three visitors, a nurse, two student nurses, a resident, and two interns. Yet there in bed lies a human being who has all the emotional problems of an office patient intensified by the certainty of serious disease and these emotional burdens to boot:

Entrapment. It's more difficult to get out of a hospital than an office, it's more troublesome to change doctors, and there's less freedom of choice in following or ignoring the doctor's orders. There's a degree of physical imprisonment even in being deprived of street clothes, to say nothing of the helplessness resulting from loss of ability to stand and walk. Although it's seldom mentioned, patients in traction spend a great deal of time wondering if they'll be trapped by fire.

Ego surrender. To be hospitalized is to place oneself back in the crib of childhood dependency. The patient is not only under orders to obey the decrees of "Papa" doctor, as applied by "Mama" nurse, he even surrenders the identity provided in the outside world by his clothing, car, street address, and occupation. Although it's combated in better medical circles, patients may be identified in the minds of nursing personnel only by location ("313, bed 2, wants something for pain"), or diagnosis ("That brain tumor is convulsing again"). Consider the ego bruises of a bank president who has his perineum shaved by an orderly and then rolls off in a split-backed nightie for a hemorrhoidectomy.

Guilt and envy. A primary reaction to illness is to feel shame for not taking better care of oneself—to feel unwholesome, a burden upon others, a piece of ugly, unhealthy corruption. With this goes aching envy of those who can walk out of the hospital at night, who are potent, free, and whole.

Over all hangs the pall of anxiety. How much will it cost? What will the outcome be? What must I give up? Who's going to take care of the business while I'm gone, and will they find someone more capable to take my place? Will it hurt? Do I have cancer?

Such a burden would be hard enough for a healthy person to bear. For the sick, depressed by weakness, locked in a cell with groaning strangers, raw-nerved from the crash of falling bedpans and the rasp of the paging system, it can be shattering.

For many patients, it wouldn't be quite as bad if they could communicate with their doctors. In the office they not only see us in privacy, they can sometimes commandeer our time by engaging a 15- or 30-minute appointment, by getting between us and the door, or by bringing up new symptoms. In the hospital the situation is reversed. The patient must await our arrival and we can walk out on him at any point in the conversation—and often do.

Somewhere, doctors have acquired a tradition of hurried hospital rounds. Perhaps it arose from the surgeon's habit of "rounding" between operations, or maybe nonsurgeons feel their income doesn't start until they arrive at the office. Maybe we're discomfited by a sense of failure in not having kept the patient out of the hospital, or perhaps we shrink from the burdens of caring for the seriously ill.

Anyway, surveys show that hospital patients suffer from lack of intimate, prolonged contact with their doctors. On the matter of discharge alone, Dr. Richard E. Alt, surgeon in chief of the Beverly (Mass.) Hospital, made a two-year study of patients and found that they had two large and often neglected areas of concern: "What are the expectations for recovery?" and "How much may I do after discharge?" Again and again it was found that these questions were *not* being voiced to the doctor because of the assumption that he would volunteer any information he thought important. Among 650 patients studied, almost half had one or more unanswered questions at the time of discharge, while almost two-thirds said they were given no specific instructions about their home care.

Happily, some of these hospital situations are improving. More private rooms are available, although there are still not nearly enough. The new hospitals are more homelike, with brighter colors and even carpeted floors. Some things are being done to reduce noise. A choice of entrees on the menu cuts down gripes about the food, and television is wonderfully distracting and entertaining for the bedridden.

All those benefits come from the administration. I think we doctors could improve our side of the situation, too.

First off, unless admission is an emergency, patients should be prepared for going to the hospital. They'll generally be uncertain and worried about three major questions:

How much? It would be a wonderful adjunct to cost-cutting and it might even uncover some accounting mistakes if every doctor got a copy of his patients' hospital bills. It would certainly help with the trouble I have in estimating the cost of hospital stays for my patients. Generally I use a figure of $50 a day for an ordinary case, but I don't really know if that's valid. Fortunately, in most cases, one can answer this question with a blithe, "Your insurance will take care of most if it," and hope that the statement is true. In any event, it's kind to let the patient know well in advance what financial hot water he's getting into, so that he can prepare to mortgage the old homestead if it becomes necessary. With hospital costs soaring as they are, people have reason to be apprehensive.

How long? This question always dogs doctors. How long will I be laid up? How long will it take to heal? How long will she live? It's common practice to duck it with a vague answer or a refusal even to hazard a guess. We've all been sensitized by the oldster who cackles for 80 years about the long-dead doctor who once predicted he wouldn't survive infancy.

But vagueness breeds apprehension, so I try to be definite, even at risk of being wrong. I can live with a mistake more comfortably than my patients can live with fear. With coronary patients, where the length of disability is standardized, it's easy to say: "You've had a heart attack. That means three weeks in the hospital and three weeks at home. You'll be back at your usual work on (date)." With diseases of less certain duration I try to sound equally definite, overestimating by 25 per cent to counteract my tendency to optimism and to hedge against the untoward. No one ever complains about getting out sooner than the estimated time. If it looks as if it's going to be longer, I give the patient a revised estimate as soon as possible, explaining why I was wrong and trying to assure him that he isn't going to be strung along by a series of such revisions.

When the patient will need to develop a new skill in order to get along with his disease, the discharge date can be a powerful motivator to learning. To diabetics I say: "You may go as soon as you can give your own insulin injection." For stroke patients it's: "As soon as you can get from your bed to the bathroom and back unaided."

What will they do? Most people, and especially those who are being hospitalized for the first time, need some understanding of what to take along to the hospital in the way of clothing and toilet articles, what the admission procedures are like, toilet arrangements on strict bed confinement, visiting hours, and other hospital rules and regulations. Some hospitals have booklets with this information, and patients faced with tonsillectomy or delivery are often given tours of the hospital in advance. But the remainder, I'm afraid, are largely left to blunder their way along. For those of us who have been around hospital routines for years, it's hard to realize how confusing and frightening they can be to the neophyte. One of the few excuses for semiprivate and ward hospital rooms is that a good roommate can do a lot to help a new arrival learn the ropes.

Of course the patient facing surgery wants to know what's coming off or out, and what he'll be like afterward. He may even want to know what's going to be done with the part of him that he's losing. We've all seen how patients treasure their gall and renal stones (when they can be pried loose from the pathologist). I once knew a mother who proudly displayed her son's appendix all over town. People should at least be given some information about pathologic exams and what happens to the things we've amputated. What to us is a corruption-filled hunk of ugly tissue is, to them, a precious piece of their former being.

People even need to know in advance where and how long their surgical scar will be. They need to know how they'll function without that precious part, especially if it's a pair of tonsils or a gallbladder or an appendix. In the way of all experts we assume that *everybody* knows the ABCs of our specialty, such as that people can function well without the aforementioned organs. But the patient often takes our silence to indicate that we're afraid to discuss the matter with him.

No matter what the malpractice risks, I don't believe in a long preoperative recital of all the things that might go wrong. If a surgeon has such poor interpersonal relations that he's afraid of malpractice suits, it would be better to send *him* to the psychiatrist than to throw his patients there with a terrifying preoperative litany of all the possible operative complications. A doctor is paid to soak up all the patient anxiety he can; I don't think it's fair to unload it on the pre-op patient. Malpractice premiums aren't that high yet, and besides we don't pay them and never will—our patients pick up that tab, as they should.

And so our patient arrives in bed. I've been taught that a person sick enough to be hospitalized deserves to see a doctor every day; many doctors go twice a day. Beyond the frequency of those visits, there's their duration and quality. We have to remember that patients don't know when we're going to pop in, so they should be given a little time to recover from surprise before we pop out.

After long practice I've schooled myself to go directly to the bedside as soon as I've picked up the chart and to do all writing and ordering there. While it's sometimes hard to write and listen at the same time, this "trick of the trade" serves several good purposes. It shows the patient how much time is spent in writing up the chart, it makes me stay in his presence, and it usually forces me to sit down at the bedside.

I recommend highly the habit of plopping into a chair. Even when one is at the bedside for the briefest moment, it gives the impression of unhurried ease. And it's surprising how much easier it is for a patient to communicate when the doctor's eyes are at his level. It was part of the old Teutonic tradition in medicine for "Herr Professor" to stand on rounds—and woe unto any hapless student who slouched or lounged in his presence. Wherever the notion came from that a hospital doctor could function only on his feet, it didn't originate with patients. Time and again, as I pull a friendly chair up to the bedside, I hear my patients' roommates say wistfully, "Gee, I wish my doctor would sit down and visit with *me* like that."

There are several things to accomplish on daily rounds beyond the obvious ones of gauging therapy. Comfort is foremost of these, so I routinely search for the little frustrations of hospital life and try to minimize them. Older people fret about bowels, so I've given up trying to teach them that intestinal intoxication is passé, and cheerfully purge them on demand. I'm also as liberal as possible in the matter of diet. Ulcer patients do very well on a general tray, I've found, and most diabetics might as well be regulated on a general diet since they're probably going to eat what they like when they leave. Soft diets, liquid diets, and such bland pap as the Sippy diet are enough to make a well man sick; I've never understood how they were supposed to make a sick man well.

I love to avoid or discontinue tubes of all kinds. I.V.'s, catheters, suction, oxygen can be lifesaving, but when they're not vital they're costly, confining, and irritating. A liter of I.V. saline contains two teaspoons of salt, four glasses of water, costs several dollars, and immobilizes a patient for two hours. Give him two teaspoons of salt by mouth, and he'll thirst for the water. The cost is nil if I take the trouble to get the salt from a salt cellar; if I order it in pill form it will cost at least a dollar. Nasal oxygen is of value only in the presence of dyspnea or cyanosis, and not always then. We don't put indwelling catheters in babies to save the nurses work, and we shouldn't do it to adults. If babies can wear diapers, so can incontinent oldsters.

In ordering blood pressure recordings or medications, I try to specify times that won't interfere with sleep. In the days of bulbar polio we used to try to bunch nursing procedures so the patient could have periods of rest. It would be nice if all patients could at least have an uninterrupted night's sleep, since it's too much to hope they'll be left alone for any moment of the day, especially in these times of virtually unlimited visiting hours.

When I find visitors at a patient's bedside (which happens as often as not these days), I try to discover whether they're casual or close friends. If casual, I get out as soon as possible, knowing that the patient isn't going to discuss anything meaningful with me but that he and the visitor will both be resentful if I'm so rude as to ask the "friend" to leave. But if the visitor is a close relative, I take advantage of his presence to close the credibility gap by telling the visitor what I want the patient to believe. As tactfully as possible I discourage the doe-eyed visitor who wants to follow me out to the hall to hear the "real" truth—while the patient lies in agony, wondering if he has cancer. Under these circumstances I turn back to the bedside and say cheerfully, "I'm sure Fred would like to hear my answers to your questions, too."

Every few days I try to go down a checklist with my patient to see if he's having bowel trouble, if the meals are hot and attractive, whether he's sleeping well, and if his call bell is being answered promptly. Bedridden patients grow fearful if their calls aren't answered with minimum delay.

Even with all this help there are still occasional patients who find it difficult to tell me their woes, so I like to read the nursing notes. Often I find surprising bits of information there about what's troubling my patients. I'd probably find a lot more if nurses could believe that all doctors always read those notes and are grateful for them.

As the time for discharge approaches I try to set a definite date and time as far ahead as possible. Once that's done I record it in the progress notes, so the nurses will be aware of it and I won't forget. That time may be relatively unimportant to me, but to the patient it's like Christmas morning to a child; he'll be properly in a snit if there's even a little delay.

Besides, going home may take a lot of coordination with the family in the way of transportation, bedroom equipment, medicine from the drugstore, and what not. I deplore the doctor who unexpectedly turns the corner, slaps down a prescription, announces that his patient is discharged, and walks out. He deserves all the telephone calls he's going to get from relatives for the next week.

Nowadays, with the team approach to care, it's equally important to warn the hospital family of impending discharge so that consultants, physiotherapists, and others can make *their* last-minute visits.

If medicines are going to be required at home, I try to get the prescription into the hands of the spouse two days ahead so she can stop by the drugstore at her convenience. For special diets, it's helpful to have the spouse sit in, too: A week is not too long to allow for instruction if the diet is at all tricky.

Pamphlets on the disease, if available, should be left several days in advance of discharge. The patient is assured that I'm going to sit down and answer any and all questions in a leisurely fashion just before he goes. Then I write down my instructions and encourage him to call by telephone any time he's having trouble.

To show him he's not abandoned, my aide calls shortly after he has arrived home and sets his first office visit. This visit will usually be a few days before the time we've set for him to return to work. He'll be fearful of that first day unless he's had recent reassurance from me, and I wouldn't want to certify him as fit for duty without a recent check. I'll also be apt to spot the occasional person who's on the verge of a compensation neurosis or an illegitimate extension of his illness into a fishing trip.

Even with the best of patient care, being hospitalized is generally a most unpleasant experience. Deductible features in hospital insurance policies may deter doctors from admitting patients unnecessarily, but I doubt that they're really necessary to deter patients from breaking down the doors to get in. Those crashing bed pans at 5 A.M. should be enough.

CHAPTER 6

Telephone Technique— Good and Bad

Marley's ghost was doomed to roam the earth encircled by chains of the cashboxes and ledgers that preoccupied him in life; the specters of most modern medicos will no doubt be festooned in telephones. When people needed the doctor in the "good" old days they had to saddle up and ride through the night to summon him. No more. The telephone has, without doubt, done as much as the doctor shortage to unravel the doctor's serenity, disrupt his family, and pre-empt his leisure.

One of the least appreciated, but most astonishing, of our services is the almost universal provision of free telephone consultation on a 24-hour, seven-day-week basis. People who wouldn't dream of calling a plumber or roofer on a holiday think little of calling their doctor from his Christmas dinner to discuss a skin rash or request a prescription refill. Patients have even been known to call the doctor at his residence merely to circumvent his cold receptionist. I've even had them call at home because they didn't want to bother me at the office!

I suppose we all have a favorite example of telephone persecution. Mine is a patient who called at 3 A.M. because he thought he might be coming down with a cold.

No one seems to know why we don't charge for our telephone services. Lawyers have to, and most other professionals find some way of charging for telephoned advice, but a MEDICAL ECONOMICS survey years ago disclosed that fewer than one in 10 doctors did, even though another survey showed that a third of our patients were willing to pay. Now that the custom is established, reversal of it would upset a lot of patient relationships. I've charged patients for phone calls on only two occasions: Neither one paid or ever returned.

The poor pediatricians suffer most. It's not uncommon for one of them to spend two hours a day on the wire. One of my acquaintances told once of taking off for an afternoon and dinner during an epidemic and returning to a list of 40 numbers to call. But in recent years, a few stalwarts have begun to charge against tradition.

A practice management question to MEDICAL ECONOMICS (5/30/66) stated that a third of the G.P.s and pediatricians at a county society meeting reported they were charging for calls and asked the consultants' opinions of the practice. While the panelists discouraged the practice, I predict a trend toward charging. If organized groups of doctors were to start the practice simultaneously, patient resistance would be minimized and an important step taken toward making the life of the practicing physician more attractive.

Meanwhile, in lieu of charging for telephone advice as a means of discouraging abuse, I've had good success with the chronic offender by insisting that he come in to be examined every time he calls, no matter how minor his complaint. He soon learns not to call unless he's troubled enough to risk the effort and expense of an office call. It must be said that *most* patients are considerate about calling. I've even been chagrined at times to hear of a man walking the floor all night in pain rather than interrupt my rest.

It must also be admitted that the over-all effect of the telephone has been beneficial to the practice of medicine and the promotion of efficiency and productive relationships. It's wonderfully comforting to perturbed parents and isolated oldsters to know that medical aid can be had at the twirl of a dial.

Doctors know apprehension, too, when there's a chance of a faulty diagnosis, or a worrisome symptom doesn't respond. In such cases an unsolicited call from doctor to patient can do wonders for both parties.

Even when he's not apprehensive, the doctor who wants to win a patient for all time might try calling when it's not expected. Sometimes I see a patient on a house call and am not entirely sure the diagnosis was right. When I report the call to my aide the next day, she puts the chart on my desk for a clinical note. As I write it, I pick up the telephone and ask how things are going. The surprise and ensuing warm gush of gratitude tell me that someone at the other end of the line is delighted to know that I care.

Most of our incoming calls are intercepted by others, as they should be. Yet we know that patients would be best satisfied if dialing our numbers always produced immediate contact with the doctor. There's inevitable frustration in having to deal with an underling, and it's compounded by postponement and uncertainty when the caller is told that the doctor is busy and will call back when he can. Rarely and inexcusably, a mother can be held home all day awaiting a return call that never comes.

Some pediatricians obviate this by setting aside stated periods when they're available by telephone; the notion has merit and could be fostered by charging a fee for all calls that come at other times.

At least, the interceptor must be carefully schooled to recognize that she is cast in the role of a foreign body and must be correspondingly gracious and helpful if she is to minimize the patient's irritation.

The formula goes something like this:

PATIENT: Is the doctor in?

AIDE: Certainly. (*Never* "Who's calling?" or "What did you want to talk to him about?" because they suggest that he's only "in" for important problems or to important people.) A pause at this point will often prompt the caller to state his business. But if not, and he proceeds with:

PATIENT: Can I talk to him?

A. AIDE: Is it about a patient? He'll want to see the chart. (This leads to a discussion of who is sick and with what.)

Or:

B. AIDE: He's with a patient. (*Never* "He's busy.") Can I help?

One way or another, it's vital that the receptionist extract the caller's name and his business before putting the call through. If the caller is a friend or relative of the patient, their relationship should be verified lest confidential information be given to the wrong party. And the patient's chart should be on the desk when the doctor picks up the telephone.

Of course, the principal reason for extracting the caller's purpose is to determine whether the matter can be handled by the aide. Many callers ask to speak to the doctor when they only wish to make an appointment. A particular pest is the salesman who takes advantage of the delicacy of our relationship by telling the receptionist that he wants to talk to the doctor on a "personal" or "private" matter. Accordingly, in our office it's a firm rule that no stranger gets through unless he states his business first.

Even when making appointments, it's vital that the aide get some notion of the caller's problem. A crass "What's the trouble?"

might meet with a "None of your business," so a diplomatic "What seems to be the trouble, so I'll know how much time to allow?" works better. It also indicates that a definite period of time is being allocated.

A doctor's family, too, must be schooled in telephone techniques. A wife who resents the intrusion of medicine upon her possession of her husband will usually communicate that feeling over the telephone. And it's important to be aware of the "little pitchers" auditing home telephone calls. The doctor who wants his sons to follow in his footsteps should realize that those sons get strong impressions of a doctor's life from his telephone reactions. If he habitually gripes when the phone rings and explodes in distemper over "stupid patients" as he bangs down the receiver, while his wife protests over the fragmentation of the family's life, embryo medics are going to abort right and left.

Some attitudes toward honesty get planted, too, when a child answers the telephone and is directed to report that father is "not in" when he is. If this sort of white lie is used, it's best to explain it thoroughly to the children and let mother do the lying. The worst faux pas of patient relationships comes when a child turns, without covering the receiver, and asks, "It's for you, Dad. Are you in?"

Home isn't the only place where others listen to our side of conversations with patients. Except in some psychiatrists' offices, it's customary to interrupt the doctor for long-distance telephone calls, calls from other physicians, and emergencies. The polite physician does not take advantage of the unwritten rule that he must be put through immediately to a colleague, but only calls when necessary and talks to the point. In the best of good manners, he leaves a message with the receptionist to have her doctor call him when free to do so and then warns *his* receptionist to put the returned call through promptly when it comes. If at all possible, he deals solely with the receptionist. But it's surprising how many referring physicians rudely insist on speaking directly to a consultant, waste his time with an involved oral case description that he'll have largely forgotten by the time he sees the patient, and then ask for an appointment. Time would be saved on both sides were the caller to delegate the appointment-making to the two receptionists and recite his history into a dictating machine.

In taking a telephone interruption, the doctor must be aware that his patient is listening and hearing only one side of the conversation (while trying to piece the whole together) and that his version of the conversation will probably be retailed to others. If possible, the doctor should either excuse himself and talk on another phone, be unrevealing in his answers, ask to call his party back at another time, or explain the conversation to the patient when it's over. In any event, he must apologize for the interruption, explain the occasion for it (since the patient will be asking himself why *he* is not put through to the doctor when *he* calls), and pick up the history at the exact point of interruption to show that he has not forgotten the thread. Even so, it may be some time before intimacy and "oneness" can be re-established.

Should the telephone be used to enhance our productivity? It takes experience and courage. Professional management experts discourage diagnosis and treatment over the telephone because of the risk of malpractice, but I must have saved patients thousands of dollars, to say nothing of thousands of hours of their time and mine, by judicious defiance of this risk.

The telephone is particularly useful in self-limited viral epidemics—the "24-hour intestinal flu," influenza, adenovirus infections, and the like that repeatedly sweep through a community. I see the first few cases in the office, check with them by telephone a few times to get the spectrum of the clinical course, and then treat all further cases by telephone.

After a few symptoms have been described I say, "I'll be glad to see you if you insist, but I think I can save you the trouble of coming in. You have the bug that's going around. You can expect to have the following symptoms in the next few days: (list them). When your temperature has been normal for two days you may return to work. I'll assume you are back at work by (date) unless I hear otherwise." (This forestalls the infrequent cheat who adds a two-week vacation to his fever and expects me to fill out his insurance papers accordingly.)

"Penicillin and antibiotics won't help you because it's a virus," I continue, and then, the most important safeguard, "*If your illness doesn't follow the course I've indicated, be sure to call me.* I'll be glad to see you at any time if you're worried or having trouble."

If the voice at the other end sounds grumpy or fearful, I surrender gracefully and make an immediate appointment. But that seldom happens if I've chanted my litany skillfully.

After the nurse has heard this recital a few times, she can begin handling the calls. By then, news of the epidemic will have diffused enough to lend support to her interposition. Even so, she should lard her talk frequently with phrases like "The doctor says . . . " and "Doctor is recommending that . . . "

The two problems I almost never attempt to treat over the telephone are skin rashes and trauma that might have fractured.

Communication by telephone, as compared with face-to-face contact, has both advantages and disadvantages. First, there's the disadvantage that fidelity is low so that voices come through with some of the more pleasant modulations and frequencies pared off. Then, too, one can't see the other person's facial expression, so that the chances of misunderstanding his mood and intent may be increased. This works two ways, however; it can be an advantage if one doesn't want to betray his inner emotions when conveying some highly charged message.

As much as the telephone annoys, interrupts, and dogs us, it has become indispensable to private practice. Our relationships to the telephone are different from those of any other worker. The problem of 24-hour availability, as promoted by the telephone, has sparked the rapid growth of groups, partnerships, answering services, emergency rooms, and salaried practice. "Getting away from the telephone" has become synonymous with la dolce vita for doctors and their families. Yet, along with the automobile, it has increased our availability, productivity, and efficiency—and thereby our earnings. Like all technical improvements, it's a mixed blessing, but this mixture is heavily weighted in favor of good for our patients. So we must be grateful to Mr. Bell despite our annoyance.

CHAPTER 7

Heading Off House Calls

One of the most important sources of doctor-patient friction—one of the areas in which we are compared least favorably with the idealized Old Family Doctor—is in the matter of house calls. The question, "Why don't you doctors make house calls anymore?" will throw any member of our clan into the gladiatorial center ring in any conversational circus. Sometimes it seems that people ask for house calls on flimsy pretexts in order to test a doctor's sincerity and availability.

Obviously, any request for a house call may ring up the curtain on a highly emotional drama, particularly now that most people have learned that we dislike making house calls, that we dislike people who ask for house calls, and that we show distaste for any conversation relating to house calls.

From the doctor's viewpoint, on a conscious level, house calls are old-fashioned, inefficient, and time-consuming. On a subconscious level perhaps we dislike them because they take us from the protective aura of our office and staff, because we are frustrated by trying to diagnose in primitive surroundings devoid of laboratory aids, and because we are resentful that house calls require our greatest physical and mental exertion while paying us at our lowest hourly wage. For some hoary traditional reason, doctors have seldom charged more for a house call than the price of an office call plus cab fare both ways. On a unit fee schedule, if an office call is 1, a house call is often 2, or, at most, 3. In relation to the time expended (and it's usually expended as overtime, since most house calls come "after hours") it should be worth 5 to 7 times the price of an office call. But rather than raise the fee, which would help to deter unnecessary requests for the service, we have increasingly refused to provide it.

This refusal and the practice of having office hours "by appointment only" have stimulated the astonishing growth of hospital emergency rooms. Here the patient can be met at the car door with a wheelchair and the assurance that immediate care is available 24 hours a day. As a result, many patients now turn to the emergency room automatically when faced by any fearful situation. Only later do they realize that they might have called their doctor first.

While the growth of these emergency room outpatient services has made medical practice more efficient and reduced the physician's loss of sleep, it has cost us some of our prestige. That's an unnecessary loss, really, because most practicing general physicians *do* make house calls. Admittedly, they do not make them wholesale as in the past, but MEDICAL ECONOMICS surveys continue to document the fact that a typical internist or G.P. makes several house calls a week.

So from the standpoint of accuracy and good public relations, there's only one answer to the provoking cocktail-hour gambit, "Why don't doctors make house calls?" That answer is, "They do. Do you know of a single instance in your own circle of friends when a doctor refused to make a house call and the patient suffered as a result? Sure, surgeons and obstetricians don't—they never did and never should—but G.P.s and internists *do*. Pediatricians don't because for a baby any car is every bit as good as an ambulance."

When patients ask, also in the abstract, "Do you make house calls?" my answer is, "Certainly, if it's necessary." There's no need to volunteer the fact that it seldom *is* necessary.

When someone calls and says, "Can you come to the house—Mother's sick?" I immediately say, "Certainly," for reassurance. But the chances are about 4 to 1 that I can get out of making that call. Here's how: After saying I'll come, my next words are, "What's the situation?" or "Maybe, if she's critical, she should go directly to the hospital to save time."

This ploy is an almost certain winner. If she *is* critical I tell them to call an ambulance and rush her in. If they say, "No, she's not *that* bad," I've at least gained time—time to put the call off until it's more convenient—and I may have opened the door to a discussion of having her brought to the office.

Almost as effective is the ploy of inquiring how long the symptom has been present. There's a fairly reliable rule that the length of time a patient waits to call a doctor equals the length of time the doctor may safely delay seeing the patient. Many exceptions occur—a patient may endure a stomachache all day and call an hour before the appendix bursts. But people with acute backaches who wait two days to call can be put off until the next day, while relatives of people with acute pulmonary edema will call immediately and with an urgency in their voices that instantly dispels any notion of temporizing.

Of course one doesn't say, "Since you've waited so long to call, I'll put you off until morning." The proper formula is, "If it's persisted *that* long it sounds fairly serious—we'd better wait until morning and investigate it thoroughly with X-rays and laboratory tests so we can get to the bottom of it."

Though it's even more cowardly, I often gain time by trying to suggest some home remedy they haven't thought of. At 5 A.M., a suggestion that ice bags be applied can stall a house call until a reasonable 7:30 A.M. Aspirin is the first thing to inquire about, foliowed by heat, baking soda (for burns, itches, gas, and heartburn), and alcoholic beverages (for pain, "nerves," and insomnia). Sometimes I've simply asked what medication was in the house and been rewarded with news of a veritable pharmacy left from previous ailments.

Naturally, this sort of stalling must be done with utmost art and delicacy, and always with the assurance, "If that doesn't work call me back in____hours (filling the blank with the number that coincides with dawn), and I'll come over."

I also get people to come to me by using the excuse of needing laboratory studies: "I'd be glad to come, but I won't be very helpful because I'll need a blood count and a urine test to determine what's going on. Why don't you bundle her into the car, drive her right up to the front door, and I'll take care of her the minute she arrives. Then I can make sure of the diagnosis and get her better faster."

Many people request house calls in order to avoid long waits in the office; a person with nausea or pain or a fever or diarrhea doesn't like to face two hours in a crowded waiting room. I duck many of these requests by assuring people that I'll see them speedily when they arrive.

On weekends and holidays, too, I try to meet patients at the office rather than go to their homes. That way they can't say I'm not willing to come out, but I don't have to locate a strange address, and laboratory facilities and records are at hand. Naturally, house call rather than office call charges are made. I usually set the time of the meeting a couple of hours hence, so that if another call comes in I can see both patients on one trip.

There are some house calls I *never* make. One is to an intoxicated patient, especially female. It's not that I hate or fear alcoholics, but that in my experience it's almost always futile; you can waste hours cajoling drunks to no avail. So after listening only briefly to the caller's slurred speech and rambling, maudlin thoughts, I say firmly, "I'm sorry, but you're drunk. Sleep it off and call me tomorrow when you're sober. I'd like to help you, and I will, but not tonight." Then I hang up.

A little foresight can avert some house calls. Asthmatics should have a supply of aminophylline suppositories in the refrigerator. Diabetics prone to sudden reactions can be supplied with glucagon and their relatives taught to inject it. People subject to gallbladder attacks or other painful seizures can be given a few narcotic tablets to have on hand. In smaller towns where pharmacists are not available at all hours, relatives can be sent to the hospital or can come to the doctor's house for medicine to ease a patient through temporary, familiar situations. In conditions characterized by vomiting, suppositories work best. Of course, relatives must understand thoroughly the rationale and technique for what may be, to them, a novel route of administration.

Sometimes, admittedly rarely, house calls can *save* time. Once I saw a young lady in an hysterical hyperventilation attack in the home where her husband and her mother-in-law hovered over me as I gave her intravenous sedation. As she reached the level of no inhibition, I asked her what was disturbing her psyche. The resulting narco-analysis audited by the two chief sources of her discontent—an overprotective mother and her passive-dependent son—did her a world of good. And I didn't have to say a word to the mother-in-law; the look on her face as I left told me she'd got the message. All in all, three people were treated in 20 minutes. It would have taken a half-dozen office visits to accomplish half as much.

Finally, there are some patients—such as bedridden invalids, cripples, people receiving terminal care at home—for whom a house call is clearly best. And after all this I must confess that, like many doctors, I rather enjoy getting into a home. Not that I'd like to make five or 10 calls a day, but I don't mind two or three a week. You really can't understand how some people live until you've been in their homes. And occasionally I pick up some diagnostic clues; poverty and poor housekeeping always make me suspect alcoholism, especially when they appear in "good" neighborhoods. But mostly I like house calls because they create a firm bond between me and my patients. Once I've made a house call, I remember the patient better as a person and he's more loyal to me. Dr. Cecil Beaton once said, "You never like a man better than when you've done something for him—and you never like yourself better, either."

CHAPTER 8

Games Doctors and Patients Play

Since the publication of Eric Berne's delightful best seller, "Games People Play, the Psychology of Human Relationships" (Grove Press, Inc., New York, N.Y. 1964), no discussion of doctor-patient relationships could possibly be complete without a discussion of medical games. Most of the "games" that follow are but variations of those described by Dr. Berne; a few appear to be new.

Berne points out that games are repetitive transactions used to avoid boredom and to give the *appearance* of productivity when, in fact, they serve to block intimacy and change. As such, they protect the status quo while giving the illusion of progress. As might be suspected, medical games flourish best among those doctors and patients who fear the risks of intimacy and among those who would rather bail boats than plug leaks. A lot of doctor-shopping goes on because game-playing patients may have to try several places before they find the proper doctor to play their particular game, or else are forced to find a new doctor when the former man refuses to play any longer.

Doctors take the lead in initiating some doctor-patient games. The game of "Take as Directed" actually starts with drug manufacturers but is enthusiastically promoted by doctors who promise a cure if the remedy is applied at the proper point in the illness. Usually that point is "at the first sign," i.e., before one can be entirely sure a bona fide attack is starting.

Required for this game are either self-limited diseases, such as the common cold, headaches, or ivy poisoning; or else cyclic diseases such as arthritis or multiple sclerosis. The doctor rakes in the chips whenever the patient improves, as is bound to happen sooner or later. But timing is all-important. In the case of the common cold, half the threatened attacks abort spontaneously, so any remedy taken "at the first sign" of a cold has a 50 per cent chance of being credited with warding off an event that wouldn't have happened. If, however, the cold materializes, it's obvious that the remedy wasn't taken "at the first sign" so the medicine gets off the hook (and the doctor as well, if it's a prescription remedy). In that event, play is continued either by giving a slow-acting remedy or by temporizing until about the seventh day, when the cold can be expected to respond to any treatment. If it doesn't, one then diagnoses a "complication" and deals a new hand of therapy. A man can get quite wealthy giving penicillin injections to people who have had their colds about a week before they can get in to see him. He can be especially successful in the medical world if he occasionally drops the remark, "It's a good thing you came when you did."

The game of "Fits" takes its title from the apocryphal tale of the old doctor who says, "I don't know what's wrong with your boy, but I'll give him some medicine that will give him fits—and I'm hell on treating fits." Among specialists, this game accounts for a lot of hobby riding. A noted allergist attained attention several years ago by proclaiming that alcoholics were attracted to their favorite beverages because they were allergic to wheat, corn, barley, or yeast. He didn't know much about alcoholism, but he was a whiz at food allergies. When a surgeon becomes proficient at a certain operation it's simply astonishing how many cases of the necessitating disease he can find.

This game is particularly attractive to the practitioner who avoids the diagnosis and treatment of emotional disorders. He'll spend hundreds of dollars trying to find some physical ailment he can treat while ignoring the obvious mental problem. He'll treat many cases of spastic colitis without treating any spastic people; tension headaches rather than husbands who are pains in the neck; and ulcers rather than obsessive, insecure personalities. On our alcoholism ward we've occasionally seen a doctor use the whole 10 days of hospitalization trying to rule out a pheochromocytoma when the hypertension was an obvious manifestation of the withdrawal state. The patient welcomes all this testing, and the topic of alcoholism somehow never comes up for discussion.

In medical centers this game is played by teachers who want typical cases of a disease to present to students. They hear only the symptoms they want when the case is first presented, and after they've lectured to students about the typical case a few times in the patient's presence, his story changes to fit perfectly the textbook pictures of the illness. In this way, medical myths such as the increase in peptic ulcers in the spring and fall can be perpetuated for generations. If an unwary student goes back to the original work-up and points out that the symptoms given at that time really could fit several other diseases as well, he is greeted with disfavor by both the patient (who wants to have a diagnosis and be a good teaching case) and the teacher, who doesn't welcome an undiagnosed or obscure case to muddy his omniscient image.

Another game to preserve our image of infallibility is "Fight the Unbeatable Foe." Here the doctor hedges by setting his patient an (for him) impossible task or regimen. Then when the patient fails, the doctor is off the hook if things don't turn out well. Here's how a typical hand might be played:

DOCTOR: Throckmorton, let me warn you again that your combination of overweight and high blood pressure makes you a prime candidate for a heart attack some day.

PATIENT: Option 1 (compliance). Yeah, Doc, I'll do better.

Option 2 (resentment). I don't eat as much as lots of other people do, and they're thin.

Option 3 (defense by attack). You look like you've put on a little weight yourself, Doc. How much do *you* weigh?

Option 4a (denial). I'm not overweight: I have a big frame.

Option 4b. Diets don't work on me.

Option 5 (fake broken wing to lure the hunter away from the nest). Did you find any signs of cancer?

. . . and so on.

The doctor's response will depend on his mood and his calculation of the odds on several possible results. He too has several options, alone or in combination, for advancing play:

1. Drop the matter. (Probably the most used.)

2. Scare the patient with a vivid description of his probable future sufferings.

3. Try to win him over with cajolery and humor.

4. Reject the patient and tell him not to return unless he mends his ways.

5. Affect nonchalance. ("I'm just giving you the advice you're paying for: Whether you follow it or not is up to you.")

6. Lure the patient with pie-in-the-sky promises of better health, longer life, freedom from symptoms, or at least a better complexion.

Of course, neither player expects any change to result from all this. On a superficial level, the doctor gains the reward of exercising a godlike power to tell others how to live their lives. His opponent gets absolution from his sins by taking his punishment in the form of confession and payment of the bill.

On a deeper level, the doctor's play is to bide his time knowing that he can't lose. When the coronary comes, he wins the game by saying, "I told you so—it's not that I'm a bad doctor but that you're a bad patient."

The patient, in the meantime, continues to enjoy his licentious life, hoping that he can postpone self-denial until the chips are down and then, by starting to take care of himself, still win the prize of healthy longevity.

In the rare instances when a patient actually *does* follow doctor's "orders," doctor is often unpleasantly surprised and frustrated. Now he can win the game only by producing the promised rewards of health, well-being, and longevity. A complexion of another color has been put on the matter.

So much for doctor games. Next, let's consider games initiated by patients, the most common of which is, "Take My Blood Pressure." In the first degree of complexity this is played by a patient's relative who is envious of the attention his kinsman is getting. As the visit terminates, the player says, "Say, Doc, while we're here, take my blood pressure, will ya?" Or he may step noisily on the doctor's scales and fumble ineptly with the weights until someone comes to help.

In the second degree, this game may involve the yearly physical exam that ranges as high as a week at a fancy resort at company expense, with mornings devoted to every conceivable test and X-ray and afternoons to golf. In addition to the obvious financial gain for the doctors and the patients' pleasure in being noticed, rested, and tested, all sorts of secondary benefits accrue. If a disease turns up (as happens rarely) the player can reap the rewards of illness while, if nothing is found, he gets reassurance that he's healthy. It's an enviable if expensive game, in which everybody wins.

Another variation of second-degree "Take My Blood Pressure" is played by the patient who says, "It (the pain, sore throat, or other presenting complaint) was pretty bad when I called for the appointment, but it's gone now." Adepts at this game know from experience that the doctor will proceed to check the place where the symptom used to be, but charge little or nothing because he isn't able to do anything productive for a symptom that no longer exists. This game can be readily broken up if the doctor has the temerity to say: "Then there's no use for me to examine you, but I'll have to charge you for the appointment time since you didn't cancel it." The trouble with breaking up games in this fashion is that the patients never come back to play anymore.

Third-degree "Take My Blood Pressure" is less benign. Here the patient chases from doctor to doctor, then from pill to pill, and finally from operating room to operating room because he can approach acceptable human relationships only from a sickbed.

"Hide and Go Seek" is a rather simple pastime. The doctor says, "What's the trouble, Mabel?" and she archly retorts, "That's what I came to find out." A more complicated form of the game appears as "I've Got a Secret." "Doctor, does it mean anything when you throw up before breakfast?" is a common opening ploy to determine how long it will be before the doctor gets to: "When was your last period?" In a game-free transaction, the exchange would be:

SHE: Doctor, am I pregnant?

HE: Do you want prenatal care, a marriage certificate exam, or an abortion?

"I've Got a Secret" is not to be confused with "Eeny, Meeny,

Miney, Moe," the game played by neurotics who present 15 symptoms in the hope that the doctor will designate one as being important enough to represent a genuine illness.

Berne describes a game, "Why Don't You—Yes, But" in which a person asks a circle of friends for advice, only to find fault with every solicited suggestion until baffled silence reigns. In medical practice this comes out as:

PATIENT: I'm nervous.

DOCTOR: Why don't you take tranquilizers?

PATIENT: Yes, but I'm afraid to get into the habit.

DOCTOR: See a psychiatrist.

PATIENT: They're too expensive, and besides they don't help.

DOCTOR: Get a new husband.

PATIENT: I love him, even if he does get drunk and beat me.

From the patient's standpoint, the object of the game is to present herself as a maiden in distress, then to stick out a foot and trip the doctor as he rushes to help her. To brighten a dull afternoon it's highly satisfying to say to such a patient, "I'm sorry but I guess there just *isn't* any help for your problem." The resulting look on the patient's face will be identical with that on a small boy's when you walk right over the purse-on-a-string he's carefully placed on the sidewalk.

In "Don't Call the Doctor," the patient (almost invariably male) really wants to see the doctor but thinks it's a sign of weakness to do so. So he walks around with one hand over his chest, leaves blood stains where they can't be missed, fails to flush the toilet, or presents some other obvious evidence of illness calculated to alarm his wife. When she makes the obvious suggestion, he replies: "Don't call the doctor. It's nothing but a little indigestion. You'd think I was having a *heart attack*, the way you carry on." *She* then marches to the telephone and calls the doctor, which is the tip-off a game is in progress. He keeps the appointment under protest and collects the payoff either way: If nothing is amiss, he gets reassurance without having admitted worry ("See, I *told* you it was nothing") and is also one up on his wife because she nagged him into the fruitless extravagance. On the other hand, if it does turn out to be the real thing, he was the stoic who endured great suffering without complaint.

The game is broken up when the doctor refuses to deal with the wife, but asks to speak directly to the husband before tendering an appointment. This puts an entirely new aspect on the relationship because if the husband now says, "It's nothing," he doesn't get to the doctor. And in any event, the wife is off the hook because she's been put out of the game.

First-degree "Don't Call the Doctor" is only a preliminary to "Take My Blood Pressure" and leads to the wife's making an appointment for her husband's yearly physical examination.

The third-degree game can be fatal when the husband plays too well and the wife postpones calling the doctor too long. Although the victory is somewhat hollow, the male still wins the role of the stoic martyr and leaves his widow with lifelong feelings of guilt because she didn't *insist* that he see the doctor in time.

"Ping-Pong" is a game characterized by alternating periods of health and disease with rewards to be collected on both sides of the net. This game is particularly favored by alcoholics, addicts, smokers, fat people, and many of the doctors who work with them. Since it's cyclic, we can enter the circle at any point. Let's say the fat lady has just come in to the doctor to *do something* about her problem. He is delighted by this invitation to play (as she knew he would be from her game-playing friends). He places her on a regimen of therapy, and the game is broadcast to all her friends, who line the field to cheer. For a variable period of time she collects all the rewards of self-approval, public acclamation, and "Take My Blood Pressure." She may even lose a little weight, although this isn't essential to the game. Finally, interest lags, appetite grows, and the other phase of the game nears. To let her move into it, almost any excuse will do: the weather, her job, "that time of the month," or the death of a distant relative. If the doctor is playing a hard game she may have to renounce him, which can easily be done on the basis of his prices, his medicine, or his personality.

Now she has a relapse, gains back all the weight (and more) that she lost, and collects all the rewards of gluttony and of pity from self and friends. When these pleasures begin to pall, she finds another rescuer, or returns to the old one, and the cycle begins again.

The offer to play is recognizable to the doctor when a patient gives evidence of working for limited or temporary goals. ("I want to lose 20 pounds"; "I want to cut down my smoking"; "Can you give me something for the shakes?—I'm just coming off a good one.") Many doctors play the game enthusiastically nowadays because it pays well, at least with obesity problems.

From the standpoint of the outsider trying to separate therapists in these fields from game players, the key question is: "How many relapses do you condone before you reject a patient?"

Variations of the game are played by diabetic children who have comas when life gets dull, epileptics who forget their medicine, asthmatics who buy a dog, and people who regularly arrange to go under the knife.

An occasional clever patient hooks me into the game of "Opposites." A lot of mental and medical therapy is based on moving against the direction of the symptom or disease. Dermatologists have joked for years about the principle, "If the lesion is weeping, dry it up; if it's crusted and dry, wet it up." It's quite obvious and reasonable that if a patient is depressed he's to be "energized," while if he's euphoric we sedate him. Accordingly, one who catches on to this game can manipulate a doctor into almost any therapy or advice he wants. I went through seven annual checkups with a businessman-patient before tumbling to the fact (when he gave a sly smile) that on each occasion he'd gotten me to encourage him to work harder by fretting over the burdens of what was portrayed as a rather average workload. Had he boasted of the amount of work he turned out I could as easily have been manipulated into advising him to "slow down."

And finally there's that innocent little game "Do *You*, Doctor?" whose purpose is to embarrass the doctor, at least, and to discredit him, at most. The patient lures the doctor into a stern lecture on the evils of some bad habit. At the proper moment the patient smiles sweetly and softly inquires, "Do *you* (smoke, drink, overeat), Doctor?" Any of his three possible answers results in checkmate. If doctor does, why can't *he* quit? If he never has, he doesn't know what it is he's asking the patient to go through. And in the unlikely event that he *used* to but doesn't anymore, he's a militant reformed sinner who gets his kicks from playing holier than thou. If he hedges or evades, the first option is assumed to be the case.

"Did *You* Ever?" is the variant played particularly on the surgical service when a patient is being encouraged to undergo something unpleasant, such as the first bowel movement after a hemorrhoidectomy or walking back to bed from a craniotomy. While checkmate is by no means as certain, the odds are all in the patient's favor if he says, "Doctor, did *you* ever have this operation?" The psychoanalyst enjoys a unique immunity from this question, because everyone knows he *has*. While this is fine for the analyst, the mind boggles at the implications of applying the principle to the rest of medical practice.

I'll leave it to the capable Dr. Berne to describe the rewards of a game-free existence. Awareness that a game exists is the science; breaking up the game without driving the patient away is the art. As for avoiding defeat in these manipulations, you can't (or at least it's very hard to) cheat an honest doctor.

CHAPTER 9

Time for the Full Life

Probably the greatest friction in the doctor-patient relationship develops from conflicts over time.

Patients would like to feel important enough to have immediate access to an unlimited supply of our time whenever they need it. When they are kept waiting for available appointment time and then are kept in the waiting room long after the appointed time expires, the heat of that friction rises. Then, if the doctor is rushed and distracted—if he is curt and cuts them off— they arrive back on the street at the boiling point. It's hard to imagine a more bruising ego-pummelling than such an encounter, because, from the patient's standpoint the doctor has said, "You are no more important to me than all my other patients, and none of my patients' time is as important as my own." Somehow, customers don't like to be put down by purveyors, especially when they're sick. For the genuinely ill, sickness with its depression and connotations of mortality is deflating enough, while the hypochondriac, hungering for tenderness and compassion, leaves feeling as though he'd been sloshed with a bucket of ice water.

Of course, from our standpoint, it's not like that at all. Busy doctors see minutes and hours as precious gems that are constantly subject to being filched. Time at work is money; time away from work is even more precious because it's so rare.

How a doctor "spends" or hoards his time tells a lot about him —about his attitude toward people, toward himself, and toward his family. Avoiding the errors of such familiar doctor types as Save-the-World Sammy, Playboy Paul, Chairman Carl, Distracted Dan, and Scientific Sam, the type I'll call Well-Balanced Willie (of which the reader and I are two rare examples), assigns his time priorities in flexible but firm fashion as follows:

First priority: Self. A sick physician serves no one well. A tired, depressed, distraught, distracted, self-pitying man can scarcely be a source of strength and happiness for others. One can care for others only to the degree that he cares for himself; he can know others only to the depth he knows himself.

The best physicians take adequate time for hobbies, recreation, exercise, social relaxation, sleep, and solitude so that they can approach their patients with pleasure.

Second priority: Family. A physician can easily use his practice as an excuse to fail his family. When he says that the diseased and dying must take precedence over his healthy children, his wife is defenseless unless she can make him see that doctors are replaceable, but husbands and fathers are not. Further, a man who is not first a loving head of the family cannot be a loving doctor. Love cannot be compartmentalized—it extends to all or to none. The physician who neglects his plebeian, unexciting hearthside responsibilities for the drama of his practice usually displays an ego-hungry need to play God rather than to be a man.

Third priority: Work, practice, patients.

Fourth priority: Community. A well-balanced, mature man cannot happily ignore the needs of his society. Of necessity, however, he will focus his energies on a few small areas where he has special interest and concern, and will have confidence enough to be able to turn down all activities that seriously threaten the first three priorities.

In medical practice, obviously, the trick is to be efficient in dispensing high-quality time to as many people as possible. But that efficiency does not necessarily lie in the assembly-line techniques practiced in many "well-run" offices. From the professional practice management view, the goal is to have as many people "seen" as possible with the least expenditure of the doctor's time and at an overhead kept exactly on the button of diminishing returns. Such a practice makes the most money, but I suspect that it's almost as frustrating to the doctor as it is to his patients.

Delegation of care to aides can be an excellent means of caring for more people—depending on the aides, the doctor, and the people. I know of a nurse who was such a warm, concerned, mother-figure that patients came to prefer her to the doctor. People took to stopping in for a cup of coffee and a visit with her when they were shopping in the area, and for years after the doctor died and she retired they would consult her by telephone at all hours. One of my solo colleagues, to whom myriads of fat ladies flock for overdoses of thyroid, is reported to have delegated so hugely that his 12 nurse-aides carry on his practice unabated while he sojourns in Florida.

But in the all-too-common instance, a patient becomes understandably hostile when he is refused a house call, then comes to the office where the nurse takes his history, the lab technician draws some blood, the nurse gives an injection, and, finally, after a long wait, the great man sticks his head in the door and impersonally announces that an infection is present and has been appropriately treated. The patient rightfully assumes that the nurse has diagnosed and treated him with minimal supervision and concern from the doctor. He leaves resenting the doctor's impersonality, angered at being treated like an unfeeling organism, and scared that the nurse doesn't know her business.

Obviously a compromise must be made. In general, the doctor who delegates the most to others must be correspondingly warmer and more personal. Advice of management consultants to add more help and delegate more procedures must be tempered at some point. For me, that point is reached when people who have a right to my time can't get it.

It seems to me that patient gripes about time fall into three categories:

1. "I had to wait too long for an appointment." Patients like to have time readily, speedily available. One of the common ways to allocate appointment time is on a first-come, first-served basis. In the early years of practice this works well, but as the practice grows, first available appointments can be pushed months ahead. The most extreme case I have encountered is that of a doctor who schedules next year's annual physical examinations on the day he does this year's because almost all the time between is taken.

Giving appointments for a far future time, especially to new patients, may be a way to limit the size of one's practice, and can certainly be an advertisement of popularity: ("My, I called Dr. G for an appointment, and they said he'll see me next October. Imagine!"). But it's not the best way. Long-delayed appointments will often be forgotten or broken and will result in a high proportion of the sterile relationships evidenced by such statements as, "I was worried about a lump in my breast when I called for this appointment, but it's gone now."

A person who calls for an appointment usually has some problem *at that moment*. Even if he asks for a routine physical examination, the call is usually prompted by some immediate fear. Simple humanity requires that his discomfort be resolved within a short time—a few weeks at most.

Too often, however, he must wait for months. Consider the unfortunate situation of both doctor and patients when the doctor is continuously booked ahead, yet always stays the same distance behind. MEDICAL ECONOMICS recently received the following plea:

"I'm a busy ophthalmologist plagued by a type of patient who's driving me cross-eyed. I wonder if anyone has figured out a way to handle him. He's the one who calls to make an appointment for a refraction, is told I can't see him for two months, and hangs up in a huff. Then, sure enough, two months later he's on the phone, ready, willing, and able to come in the next day because 'you said you could see me.' But he didn't make an appointment the first time, so he's back at the end of the line—and doesn't like it.

"I wish there were some way to handle him and all the other types who want to talk, who must see me before leaving for Europe tomorrow, and who otherwise make my appointment book look like a bombed-out ballpoint pen factory.

"M.D., Pennsylvania"°

Somehow this doctor must catch up, and then stop booking two months ahead. If he stays steadily two months behind, he is simply seeing old appointments at the same rate that new ones are made; the two months' lag represents no advantage to him and is a distinct frustration to his patients. Any physician whose appointments get booked even *one* month ahead should promptly begin to limit his practice by one or more of the methods suggested in Chapter 18. Only doctors and dentists schedule appointments months in advance, and it's an inefficient and inexcusable custom.

Then too, booking appointments far ahead has an interesting effect on a doctor's practice. If he is a specialist who depends on

°March 6, 1967.

referrals, other doctors will gauge his popularity and success by the lag in his appointment time. For example, suppose I discover the possibility of a disease in a patient's eye. Knowing how much apprehension even the simplest flaw in vision arouses, I'll want to get the issue settled as soon as possible—ideally, for me and my patient, that same day. The only ophthalmologists who will be apt to have appointment time in the next few weeks will be the very old, semiretired men whose medical skills are slipping, or one of the recent arrivals in town. When my secretary tells me that the young man who came to town four years ago is booking my office referrals one month hence, I'll probably stop sending patients to him and start using a newer man. The first consultant won't miss my business much because he's already decompensating for time, but, subtly, the character of his practice will change because he will now see fewer acute cases and fewer referred cases: From now on, most of his work will be with previous patients who are returning for regular and routine care. He'll be making more money and life will be less hectic for him—but his practice will be less exciting and challenging.

Thus there is youth, middle age, and old age in a practice, and the gray hair and wrinkles can be seen in the appointment book.

But a practice can be kept young for a while, if the doctor desires it, by providing time reserves to ensure that referred and acute cases can always be seen in a few days. If there's anything a referring physician appreciates, it's prompt, efficient service. And if there's anything a worried patient appreciates, it's the words, "Come right along—Doctor will see you as soon as he can after you get here."

2. "Why does he make an appointment and then keep me waiting for hours?" It's not so much the discomfort of sitting with a tired magazine that bothers—the chances are that some of the loudest complainers would be doing pretty much the same thing if they were home. What matters is, first, a broken contract: "The doctor agreed to meet me at 1 P.M. I kept my word,

but he's broken his." Then there's the obvious insult: "He thinks it's all right to keep *me* waiting because his time is so *much* more important than mine." Finally, there's the frustration and uncertainty: "Was this delay really necessary? How much longer is it going to be?"

A practice that is habitually off schedule tells me that the doctor-manager has one of four emotional problems:

- He gets ego-satisfaction out of a full room of people waiting for *him*.
- He's too self-centered to care about other people's feelings.
- He's so insecure that he tries to please everyone.
- He's sadistic.

If those choices seem harsh, see if you can list any others. You may want to add to the list those doctors who apparently have a congenital indifference to time. I know one such doctor who schedules appointments by having his receptionist tell everyone for the whole afternoon to arrive at 1 P.M. He and his wife are so notoriously late for parties that hostesses take care to invite them at least an hour earlier than the other guests. But he never misses an airplane.

And don't put the blame on inefficient aides. In my experience, whenever one of my employes has packed the schedule to overflowing it is because she was trying to meet *my* desire to help too many people.

Obviously, giving patients adequate, high-quality, uninterrupted time involves skilled scheduling. More than that, it requires that the doctor possess a dedication of the sort that rubs off on his aides. Here are some schedule precepts that serve me well:

A. Time is not expandable. "Squeezing" extra people into a full schedule means that the schedule will run late the rest of the day or that some sick Peter will be robbed to make room for Paul.

B. A schedule is a contract between the patient and the office.

If the patient is on time he has a right to expect that the office will be.

C. "Work expands to meet the time allotted to it." That's why a schedule may often run behind but seldom runs ahead. But it also means that the allotment of more time to a task, up to a point, will encourage thoroughness and a more relaxed approach.

D. Any amount of time may be given to an individual. So long as that time is spent productively, he'll be willing to pay for it.

As everyone knows, however, even the best-run offices occasionally run behind. When that happens, there are several lubricants to reduce the friction. In my practice, when we get 15 minutes behind, I try to greet each new arrival personally and explain why and how much we're running late. At the 30-minute delay point, we offer another appointment. If delays stretch any longer, my secretary gets on the phone to head off someone further down the schedule who has not yet left home.

3. "When I finally do get to see him, he rushes me so much I forget half I want to say—and even then, he doesn't seem to listen." This common comment is a criticism of both the quantity and quality of time received. There *are* some patients who steal time by nonproductive rigmarole, but the usual source of this conflict is, I think, a difference between the amount of information the doctor needs and the quantity that the patient feels he should impart.

There's a medical school shibboleth: "Listen to the patient—he's giving you the diagnosis." That isn't true very often in office practice. Mostly, he's giving a lot of unrelated and unimportant symptoms he's noted and carefully rehearsed or written down. It isn't that he's trying to get more than his money's worth; he simply wants us either to treat each symptom or to reassure him that it's harmless. Our ability to evaluate his various aches and pains and queer sensations is, of course, precisely what he's paying us for.

Even so, when a patient makes an appointment to talk about

headaches, I find myself getting irritated if he wanders off into a discussion of his fallen arches. I have to remind myself that, from his standpoint, it's smart to unburden all his medical problems while he has my attention. *My* problem is that I'm all clenched to spot a brain tumor, while "headache" simply happened to be at the head of his list when the receptionist asked what he wanted to see me about.

To be sure, doctors are often so pressed that they're in a hurry from morning to night. Yet I think people are attracted to relaxed doctors, as well as relaxed TV performers. As Dr. Michael J. Moore has pointed out, the trick is to conceal from the patient the fact that we *are* hurrying—to cultivate the habit of appearing relaxed, so that he won't *know* he's being hustled. One of my most effective devices is to record a patient's every complaint, without comment. When he's finished I ask, "Is there anything else?" Then I inquire further into the one or two complaints that have merit and ignore the rest. Nine times out of 10, transferring a symptom from his paper to mine satisfies his need.

Insofar as possible, I take down his words verbatim. Some hold that a doctor should take only the briefest notes and later dictate the history for typing. But I think there's therapeutic merit in having my patients see me writing furiously as they talk—obviously I'm taking *all* their complaints seriously.

A lot of thought has been devoted to ways of saving doctors' time but it's rare to see any attention given to saving patients' time. I've found several time-savers for patients that require no great sacrifice on my part. The biggest one, of course, is to work by appointment and to be waiting for the patient when he arrives. Next in order is to handle everything possible by telephone. In some offices a patient comes once for examinations and returns a second time for reports—which are almost always normal. I spare him the second visit by having my secretary call and tell him the results. We never set up an appointment just to give reports. If I'm pretty sure a man's X-rays are going to show an ulcer, I give him his instructions and prescriptions on the initial visit, before the X-rays are taken. Then when I call to tell him the X-rays are positive we can chat about his progress and save him another visit.

When new diabetics have been started on treatment, I call every few days to get reports of urine tests. Only when I've adjusted the insulin dosage by telephone to clear the urine of sugar does he need to spend the time (and money) to get a blood sugar.

Since we do our own ECGs, those reports are ready before patients leave the office. When diabetics come for routine checks, they are seen; the blood sugar is drawn; then I call later in the day to give results, set any change in insulin dosage; and make the next appointment. Reports on elective X-rays are given by telephone. In the case of emergency X-rays, the patient goes from my office to the radiologist down the hall and then returns to me about the time the radiologist is calling with a "wet reading" on the film.

While a patient is in the office we try to keep him busy every minute. In some practices the doctor tries to keep three or four examining rooms occupied. That means one patient with the doctor, one dressing or undressing, and one or two undressed and wondering whether it's going to be five or 50 minutes before someone pops in the door. With examining tables as uncomfortable as a marble slab, they'd be better off waiting in the waiting room—and best off waiting at home until the doctor is ready to give them his undivided attention.

But can every doctor afford to permit that? What about the man who feels that his patients won't pay more than $7 for an office visit, so that he can't make a reasonable profit unless he sees four people an hour? In my experience, patients are happy to purchase a full hour of a doctor's time at the going rate if the quality of that time is good—far happier than they are with a lower price for less time of inferior quality.

The time a physician allots to his patients determines the type of patients he sees, the effectiveness of his relationships, the size of his practice, and, to some extent, the amount of leisure he enjoys. Time spent with patients is also a measure of a physician's ability to relate to people.

For example, a man who sees 300 patients a week isn't going to have time to know very much about any of them. He will treat symptoms on a superficial basis and run an operation that is something like an Army dispensary. He'll spend his "on call" evenings and weekends at home on the telephone, because of the many people who depend upon him for medical care. And I can't imagine how he remembers who they all are when they call him.

He will need many more hospital beds than the doctor with a normal practice, and will tend to put people in the hospital more readily because he doesn't have time to study them thoroughly in the office. Generally, he runs increased risks of malpractice, and is chronically tired and frustrated.

The physician who sees 65 patients a week, by contrast, will have fewer emergency calls and will tend to know a great deal about his patients as people. Because of his close relationships and despite the much larger bills he submits, he will hear fewer complaints about fees.

Many doctors in general practice rationalize that they could not get patients to pay $25 to $30 an hour for their services. In truth, they would be uncomfortable spending an hour getting to know a patient's problems that intimately, and they don't believe people will pay just to talk to a doctor—that they'll pay only for procedures performed upon them. All I can say is: "Try it." Schedule one 60-minute period each day for one patient to be seen without interruption and do the kind of work-up medical students are trained to do. Then charge as much as you do for any other hour of office work. After a few months, review the experience from the standpoint of income and satisfaction and determine whether you wish to continue.

The difference between a wonderful day and a terrible day in my practice is often the difference between being a half hour ahead of schedule or a half hour behind. The best way to enjoy being a doctor, for me, is to allot a little more time for each task than it takes. I think of it as being generous—to myself, my family, my aides, and my patients. You can't beat a policy that makes *everybody* happy.

CHAPTER 10

Are You Sure You're Charging the Right Fees?

It's not the province of this chapter to dissect fee schedules and collection techniques, but rather to discuss the important ways in which the exchange of money for service affects the doctor-patient relationship.

From the patient's standpoint, buying a medical service is worse than buying a pig in a poke: "Emptor" doesn't get much chance to "caveat." Despite all kinds of fancy signs inviting patients to discuss medical fees, it's seldom done unless the doctor brings up the subject. Besides, it wouldn't do much good, because a patient has little way of gauging the value he receives. When a television repairman fails to fix the set, he doesn't get paid because, short of near-demolition, there's no such thing as an irreparable set. A veterinarian may not charge more than the replacement value of a farm animal, dentists pull and replace bad teeth, and lawyers often work on contingency. By contrast, it's almost unique to medicine that results are never guaranteed and, indeed, the worse those results are, the more costly the treatment is apt to be.

What extraordinary faith people have in us to let us set our own contracts! And now insurance carriers and the Federal Government are displaying some of that same trust. In some instances they've discovered it's cheaper to give the doctor what amounts to a signed blank check than to use fee schedules.

This return to the pre-Blue Shield era of individual fees will restore, at least to the doctor in solo practice, a chance to use fees to meet his own psychological needs. For example:

1. The need to play Robin Hood (otherwise known as robbing Peter to pay the rent). By charging rich people more, one "gets even" with those he subconsciously hates or envies. He can excuse his actions by saying that rich people demand more service, or that their care places a heavier burden of responsibility on the doctor's shoulders, or that the practice is necessary to subsidize free care for the poor.

A doctor can next collect a reward on the other side of the street by reducing fees to the indigent. He then warms his hands in the glow of his own magnanimity—so long as he does not reflect that it was the wealthy patient and not the doctor who made up the difference.

The obvious pitfalls of trying to guess a patient's economic status, of believing that the wealthy patient will be unaware of his higher fee or that the poor patient will be grateful, have made this practice wane in late years. That mythical paragon of medical practice, the old family doctor, is said to have carried it out with considerable élan, aided by his intimate knowledge of the economics of his small community. (But then, it seldom mattered *what* he charged since he is reputed to have been above the nasty practices of billing and collecting fees anyway.)

2. The need to buy friends by giving cut-rate services. An older doctor told me when I started practice that I shouldn't be

excessively concerned with my fees, since they would tend to rise and fall with the demand for my services. To some extent, he was right, at least in the early days of my practice when there were unfilled hours in the schedule. There is a close relationship between the doctor's confidence and the fees to which he feels entitled. If his confidence is sagging because the phone has stopped ringing or he has had a series of unfortunate cases, his fees will tend to droop. Conversely, the feeling that he is skillful, sought after, and sagacious will cause them to rise.

A physician with depressive tendencies will be wise to turn his fee setting over to his receptionist and management consultant. Contrary to the usual laws of economics, lowering medical fees can decrease demand for his services. Within reasonable limits, the public, for want of better criteria, tends to judge a doctor and his services by the fees he charges, leading to conversations like this:

A: I go to Dr. X.

B (admiringly): I hear he's awful high priced.

A (proudly): He certainly is!

The economically shy, insecure doctor may underprice himself into self-perpetuating financial atrophy, while the extrovert and the hypomanic whiz by in Cadillaceous self-esteem. In fee setting, nothing succeeds like success.

3. The need to punish or reward a patient. A given patient may behave badly in his doctor's eyes, either overtly, by demanding favors or refusing to follow directions, or covertly, by failing to get better. In these instances fees may come up a bit. Conversely, the patient who improves spectacularly and the one who is extravagant in his praise of the physician may get off lightly.

Horace Cotton, the well-known practice management consultant, writes of a "cheerful fee"—one that is charged and paid without gloom on either side. Patients have psychological stakes in fees, too. There will seldom be gloom from the side of the patient who is convinced that his doctor cares for and about him. A patient who trusts his doctor trusts him not to overcharge. When a patient complains about a fee it is almost invariably a sign of anger toward a physician who failed to understand and meet his emotional needs. If that anger does not blow the safety valve of a protest over the fee, it may explode in a malpractice suit. Lesser forms of dissatisfaction may be expressed by delaying payment for several months: It's a common aggressive reaction for a patient to ignore statements until threatened with stronger attempts to collect, at which time he protests about the quality of services rendered three to six months previously.

In checking on his "art" as a doctor, it's a good idea for a physician to be aware of his collection percentages. Assuming reasonable fees and good collection techniques, if he collects less than 90 per cent of his bills he's probably not intimate enough in patient relationships.

Whenever there is a protest over fees, he should be informed. He should then review the chart and discuss the matter personally and reasonably with the patient. (Few patients protest fees in person, so this conversation will probably take place over the telephone.)

He will be wise to get a stranglehold on his emotions, and he will be lucky if he's in a happy frame of mind when faced with such a challenge to his integrity and confidence. If he reacts with bluster, denial, or ire he will probably not only lose the whole fee as well as the patient, but may well face a protest to the medical society or a malpractice suit in retaliation.

He must stop to reflect that people have to be pretty hurt and disappointed to call and complain, so feelings on the other side of the line probably run high, wide, and ugly. He can be grateful that he is being given a chance to change his fee, since many patients will simply not come back, or will give the doctor his first inkling of their dissatisfaction by taking one or more of the punitive measures mentioned above.

His alternatives are to: (1) stick to his guns, (2) cut the fee somewhat, or (3) write it off altogether. Of these, the second is nearly always most prudent.

Failure to change the fee will risk driving the patient to more unpleasant actions, while throwing in the entire fee sponge is an aggressive and immature act that will certainly drive the patient away permanently. It may also lead him to suspect that the fault in his care was even greater than he surmised.

The wise physician begins by thanking the patient for taking the trouble to inform him of his displeasure and then offers assurance by words and tone of voice, that he is a reasonable man and is eager to adjust the matter to the *patient's* satisfaction. Hudson's department store in Detroit has built its reputation in part on the fact that it has never protested a customer's complaint; even when worn goods or materials obviously purchased in other shops are returned, the adjustment is always made to the customer's complete satisfaction. The rewards in goodwill outstrip the cost. So it is in medicine. The doctor should hear the patient out without interruption, urge him to ventilate thoroughly any other complaints he may have, apologize sincerely, and then ask the patient what he considers to be a reasonable fee. If there is a complaint that might be worthy of a malpractice suit, one does not, of course, agree with the patient: The apology should be for failing to give satisfaction, *not* for failing to practice good medicine.

The smoke from such a fee explosion may pollute the poor doctor's atmosphere in several ways:

1. He will feel that he lost a fight not of his choosing, and retreated from an opponent of lesser size without striking a blow.

2. He may fear that the word of his weakness will spread, and encourage others of his clientele to try for reduced rates.

3. He may resent all patients in general and this one in particular for robbing him of his godlike position above error and criticism.

Mature reflection will assure him that it takes a big man to walk away from a fight, that people seldom boast about winning transactions of this sort, and that he should be grateful for a reminder that he is sometimes imperfect. A mature, well-adjusted, secure individual accepts criticism well.

A fee cheerfully charged and paid can be a wonderful adjunct to patient-doctor relationships. The reader is referred to the chapter on doctors and doctors' wives as patients for a discussion of the deterioration in relationships that may arise when *no* fee is charged for services of obvious value. The interposition of a third party, such as a clinic or hospital that collects fees and hires doctors on a salary, blunts those relationships, too. I became aware of this in my own case when I left residency to enter private practice, then spent two years as a physician in the military before returning to practice. During my periods on salary I was delighted when patients failed to show up for appointments and I was unhappy when the schedule was full, while in private practice my reaction was just the opposite.

Doctors on salary are apt to regard stupid or demanding patients as "crocks," while private practitioners are likelier to regard these same individuals as lovable eccentrics, at least so long as they pay their bills.

One of the reasons we are reluctant to market the service of house calls is that we have seldom charged the $25 to $30 that would enable us to make them cheerfully. Our failure to charge enough has made us resentful of being called upon to give this service (except to very special patients), with the result that the public feels hurt and angry because we reject them or yield grudgingly when they want us most.

For these reasons I find that I practice the most intimate,

cheerful, and satisfactory medicine when I charge more—not a lot more, but just a little more—than the going rate in my community. This shows my patients that I have confidence; it gives them a feeling of getting better-than-average care; and most important, it makes me hump to provide services that will justify those fees.

When I find myself resenting a patient's demands, I raise my charges to him until I'm happy to meet his demands. Then he can have a cheerful rather than a resentful doctor, and that's healthy for both of us.

So much for the philosophy of fees. Here are some specific fee management principles for maintaining good relationships, culled from experienced practice management consultants and MEDICAL ECONOMICS surveys of patient attitudes:

1. Fees over $20 for people of average means should be discussed in advance by the doctor. This is particularly important in surgery and obstetrics.

The schema for this discussion is: "My usual fee, and that of the majority of the doctors who do this procedure, is $_____. This charge covers_____, _____, and_____. It does *not* cover unusual complications that might arise. You can expect hospital and laboratory fees to run about $_____. If you have insurance, we will help you get all the aid from that source to which you are entitled. Is this arrangement satisfactory?"

All the figures are then written down in duplicate and placed not only in the doctor's file but in the patient's hands, because there's at least a 40 per cent chance that, under the duress of the impending operation, he'll forget or misinterpret what was said.

2. The highest collection ratios are enjoyed by those doctors who charge going rates, who render good service, who use collection techniques that help their patients pay promptly (when gratitude is at its peak), and who itemize all charges intelligibly.

3. The full extent of services rendered should be explained to

the patient. A commonly heard gripe is: "He called in a consultant who only spent 10 minutes with me and charged me $50." Or worse, "Some strange doctor showed up and asked a lot of questions and then sent me a bill." Such difficulties could be avoided if the referring doctor would offer some explanation of why he's calling in a consultant and if the consultant would—by such devices as reading the chart and writing his notes at the bedside —give the patient some idea of how much time he spends on the case.

(Anesthetists have a particularly difficult time convincing their debtors because, if they do a good job, the patient should be almost totally unaware of the service rendered.)

It is relatively easy to avoid friction over fees between individual doctor and individual patient by use of these precepts.

Much harder is the task of promoting better feeling on these matters between the general public and doctors as a whole. Because we're in a sellers' market and because we work an average 60-hour week, we're shamefully rich. If we could charge what is needed to attract more youngsters to medicine and if we could deny care to people who can't meet our charges, we'd be even richer.

There's a lot of ambivalence surrounding our incomes: Our patients want to go to expensive doctors, but they don't like large fees; they believe that expensive medicine must be good medicine, but complain of high doctor incomes. We doctors are ambivalent, too: We don't charge for telephone calls and then resent people who phone for medical advice; we'd like to take the best care of everyone without regard to cost, but we oppose Federal subsidization of health care. MEDICAL ECONOMICS surveys show that doctors place "income" well down the list of sources of satisfaction from their specialties, but they also show that the highest-paid specialists are the most satisfied. And we feel guilty that the average doctor earns more than a medical school dean or the average state governor while we campaign vigorously for higher fee schedules.

Moreover, we're almost licked from the start in trying to keep the public happy about medical bills. It's common to compare the amount the public spends on liquor and tobacco with expenditures for health care, but I think this is like trying to compare marriage and measles. When people buy a new car or dress or television set, they feel they're ahead of the game, but a doctor at best just gets them back where they were before they got sick.

We must face the unpleasant fact that we are in the repair business, which means people aren't going to be happy about having to call us. People like to buy a new car, but they don't like to pay for repairs on it; they like a new washing machine, but they don't like to have to call a plumber to stop a leak; they'll cheerfully pay several hundred dollars for a television set and carp when it costs $25 to have it fixed.

Further, illness is unexpected and unplanned. When a person buys a car he usually knows about what he's able to pay, and he plans the date of purchase far ahead. Illness strikes without warning and almost always upsets plans.

A further source of distress over our fees is that much of our work is intangible. People have to pay fees to anesthetists, radiologists, surgical assistants, and pathologists they don't even know. They can't appreciate their surgery deeper than the scar, and unless they're the President of the United States they may not even be able to display *that* in public. There *are* some tangible benefits in being rid of pain, but very few in receiving advice on how to avoid a painful illness in the future. And we're in one of the few occupations where people are charged just for talking with us.

Because we're unable to replace many parts, we're seldom able to restore our customers to being as good as, or better than, new.

Most illnesses leave some scar, some irreparable residual, so we can rarely produce 100 per cent customer satisfaction.

And then, we and criminal lawyers are often the only vendors who have to run up a bill at the one time when the breadwinner of the family is unable to work, which puts us in the position of kicking a man when he's down.

With all these handicaps it may well be that what some of us call "socialized medicine" will do more to improve our customer relationships than can presently be imagined. If so, we could use the help—we've certainly made enough enemies by opposing it.

But if the time does come when all our fees are paid by third parties, I hope they'll preserve our fee-for-service right and not put us all on a salary. I need the feel of charging directly to bring out the best in me.

CHAPTER 11

The Management of Problem Patients

Let's face it: Being human, we all encounter certain types of patients we simply can't stand. It's a good thing that we don't all reject the *same* types, though, or some people would never be able to find sympathetic care. As house officers discover, one doctor's "crock" may be another's "nice little old lady." The result is a sorting out of difficult patients until each finds a physician who tolerates his particular quirk. Dr. A will attract selfish, wealthy socialites; Dr. B will be burdened with the poor and uneducated; Dr. C will cater to fat, nervous ladies who expect lots of injections and tranquilizers; Dr. D will care for a lot of schizophrenics.

The patients a doctor attracts and rejects tell a lot about him. I've learned a lot about myself by asking, "Why is it that I dread seeing Mrs. Murgatroyd's name on the appointment schedule?" Usually, the answer is that she threatens to take something away from me. More often than not, it's my precious self-esteem.

In the early days of practice, my self-confidence was shaky

from youth, inexperience, and the abrasion of the medical training process. It didn't take much to threaten me, so I disliked many different kinds of people. I've seen the process in many other medical neophytes. While understandable, it's unfortunate, because it's when a man's practice is new that he most needs to attract all kinds of people. Later, when he's confident enough to cope with problem patients, he's apt to be too popular to have time for them.

At first, I assumed that people with prickly personalities were best handled in a strictly professional manner and were to be accepted as the inevitable flotsam that floats in to a new doctor's office. With such an attitude on my part, it's not surprising that many of them floated right back out again—which didn't do much for my self-esteem either.

The breakthrough came during the honeymoon era of cortisone for arthritis. Prior to that time, in common with most doctors, I hated to see an arthritic coming because treatment was so unsatisfactory. Then came cortisone, and, until the side effects became apparent, I wished I could treat every arthritic in town because the results were so brilliant and the patients so grateful.

That experience taught me that I only liked people I could help—because they made me feel more of a doctor and because I needed to feed on their gratitude. It's only human to want to be successful and to avoid lost causes; observe the surgeons clustering at the bedside of the preoperative cancer patient and how they scatter from him when laparotomy has disclosed metastases.

Then it became obvious that the same rejection of patients with hopeless physical disorders was dogging my treatment of people with unfortunate personalities. Soon I was trying to change myself as well as my problem patients, so we could enjoy each other. In handling some types of difficult people, better understanding of myself is the major requisite; in other cases it's worthwhile to help the patient change, so that he can be a more acceptable person not only to me but to others and himself. Usually we both change. Understand, I haven't achieved the ability to solve *all* my problem patients—a lot of challenge will have gone out of medicine if ever I do—but here are some of the techniques and insights I've gained so far.

One of my common problems is the new patient who is hostile before I've given him any reason to be. This always suggests the well-known phenomenon of displacement. If the patient doesn't see me as a father he hates, he may see me as an extension of his nagging wife, or as a symbol of the frailty and illness that threaten his masculinity.

In the old days I'd have been hostile right back, and our relationship would have been brief. Now I've learned to enjoy the challenge of breaking through that angry shell.

First, his anger doesn't threaten me if I realize he doesn't have any reason for it. (This security on my part only arises when I know that our appointments are running on time and my aide is cordial.)

So I smile at him—not a crooked smile or a derisive grin—just a big, broad, friendly smile to let him know that I'm comfortable with his anger. Sometimes, that's enough. As the interview progresses the tension will relax, and we'll part friends.

If my failure to assume the defensive antagonism he anticipates *doesn't* suffice, it's time for confrontation: "I sense that you are upset and angry this morning. At first, I thought you might be angry at me, but then I realized you don't know me that well. Do I remind you of someone?"

If the identification is made it's worthwhile to encourage ventilation of his feelings toward the hated person and then to help him to understand his dislike, without necessarily siding with him on the issue. As a further step, I try to help him to understand the behavior of that other person. If a man can understand why his father or his boss behaves as he does, he'll probably stop disliking that person, and then he'll stop disliking me as a representative of that person.

Another problem I encounter frequently is the patient who frustrates me when I find he's not giving me the whole truth and nothing but the truth. Actually, it's probable that very few of our clientele are perfectly candid, or that we doctors are any less free of deceit when we consult colleagues about our own illnesses. Sometimes patients are embarrassed to tell us of intimate problems; sometimes they fear we will judge or reject them.

If it's important to get the whole story, reassurance that one is not going to be judgmental, followed by smiling confrontation, is helpful. So is taking time to win the patient's confidence before coming back to the point. The word "confidence" comes from "confide"; one confides to another in whom he has confidence or trust. A physician who fails to penetrate his patient's secrets has failed to inspire confidence. In turn, we may reject the reserved or secretive patient because he threatens *our* security and tells us covertly that he does not find us trustworthy.

Nonverbally he communicates that an area of delicacy, shame, or embarrassment is near. On both sides there may be ambivalence about getting this material out or suppressing it. But the productive physician will push on, recognizing that material painful enough to provoke such an uncomfortable reaction may well be an important facet of his patient's primary disease; he may be close to "cracking" the case.

Several techniques can be useful. Dr. Thomas P. Hackett, psychiatrist at Massachusetts General Hospital, suggests that the doctor guess at the very worst things he can conceive: "Have you had intercourse with one of your brothers?" . . . "With an animal?" This, he says, eases the strain of confessing lesser matters. He also finds it helpful to ask the patient to repair to the waiting room with paper and pencil to write what cannot be spoken.

A rare means of getting a patient to confess is the technique long used by police officers. When they catch two men in a crime, you'll recall, it's common to separate them and then tell each that the other has confessed. Similarly, a doctor can sometimes hint that he already has the knowledge he needs. This can be risky business, needless to say. For example, say a man comes in with obvious signs of alcoholism but denies drinking to excess. Since it's known around town that I'm interested in alcoholics, I might be able to say, "Several people have been concerned enough about your drinking problem to discuss it with me over the past few years—you don't know it but I've been laying bait for you all over town. I'm glad you've come; I've been looking for you because I think I can help you." Note that the victim is given no concrete information he can contradict and no names of people he can hate. If he counters with, "My wife has been talking to you," I answer with a question: "Why should she do that? Has your drinking been bothering her?"

My favorite technique for the embarrassed patient is to say, "From the way you're hesitating, I gather we're getting close to your real problem. You know that I'm a doctor, that anything you say will be confidential, and that you can't possibly tell me anything I haven't heard dozens of times before—so go ahead: Out with it."

Then I carefully place my note pad and pencil aside to indicate that I'm not going to write down this part of the history (although I *will* put it in the record after the patient has left) and sit silent. Silence is a potent weapon to force the patient to communicate.

At times the doctor-patient relationship may be such that it would be unwise to uncover guilty secrets. One could hardly expect his golf partner to confess an illicit love affair, or a neighbor to seek help for sexual perversion. I have occasionally had patients transfer to my care because they had come to know their old doctor on such a personal basis they could no longer "level" with him. And that is by all odds the best solution to these quandaries: Encourage such people to go to a stranger.

Recently an old maid whom I've succored over the years developed panic attacks which she felt were physical in origin. I was able to convince her that they were emotional, and she was able to hint that there were "sexual problems," but neither of us was willing to discuss the obvious coincidence of her attacks with the recent presence of a young female companion in the house. When she suggested psychiatric consultation I eagerly agreed. She called later to report that she had been able to tell "a stranger" some things she hadn't wanted to tell me, "because you have become such a close friend."

Dr. Hackett also suggests the possibility of an oblique approach in such cases. When the physician is pretty sure of the source of his patient's guilt he may discuss such problems in the abstract. Accordingly, in the sample of my old maid I could have said, "Some people get palpitations and feelings of fearfulness because they have sexual yearnings that society would disapprove, but they would rest easier if they knew how common these impulses are and realized that there's a wide gulf between having an impulse and submitting to it."

Yet another technique, when one guesses what the source of the embarrassment may be, is to bring it up at the end of the examination. If the doctor senses that his patient is concerned about cancer or syphilis for example, he may wait until the end of the exam and casually include in his summary of findings the information that such a condition was not found. If the patient responds with a long "Whew!" of gratitude and relief, he will be signaling that he'd like to stay on the subject and have the doctor discuss the source of his phobia.

A more common difficulty is the loquacious patient who interrupts productivity by needless details, meandering thought, or refusal to listen to the question asked. It will be important to listen quietly for awhile to determine whether this represents a form of embarrassment, the chaotic thought processes of psychosis, mental deficiency, a cover-up for deafness or senility, a lonely hunger to visit with an understanding ear, or simply the product of an undisciplined mind.

A nonverbal expression of impatience is the usual first defense. One can "cut in" with short, direct questions in a sharp tone of voice, look stern and unhappy, drum his fingers, or look at his watch.

If this fails, smiling confrontation may work: "See here, I asked you if you had headaches and you're telling me about the pain in your side. Let's get through with one subject before we get on to another, or you'll have my notes all fouled up. We'll get to your side pains later."

When a patient starts off with a long meandering preamble it's sometimes productive to interrupt with, "What's your problem— tell me in one sentence." While this might seem brutal to another type of patient, it's common to see no emotional reaction in the compulsive talker, or even a reaction of relief that some limits have been set.

That brings up the subject of disciplining patients. One cannot love an untrained child; discipline is no less essential to productive adult relationships. Experienced, confident doctors seldom hesitate to train their patients to behave acceptably. The techniques should be dignified and kindly and should be kept in "the here and now." One does not dredge up long-past unpleasantnesses nor impugn the patient's motives or character, but simply tells him how his actions affect the ability of the doctor to know and like him.

For example, rather than let a patient run up such a bill that it becomes impossible for him to continue as a patient, I might say smilingly, "Ralph, my accountant says that your bill is getting out of hand. Sooner or later that's going to make it hard for me to serve you as willingly as you and I would both like."

A particularly good point at which to apply discipline comes with the patient who apologizes first and then goes ahead and transgresses.

"I'm sorry to call you on your day off doctor, but——." If the patient has done this before, the proper answer is not, "That's all right," but rather, "I don't mind being called if you're in pain or if you think it's a real emergency, but if you *could* put off your calls until my regular hours I'd prefer that you do so. Besides, when you call me at home I don't have your records available, so I can't give you as much help." Or, "I'm sorry, but I don't recall just which medicines you're taking. This doesn't sound too serious at the moment—suppose you call me at the office tomorrow and we'll work it out." (More intimate variant: "I'll make a note and call you from the office tomorrow.")

Sometimes wives and secretaries can be encouraged to train patients when doctors are temperamentally unsuited to the task. A wife can say, "The doctor is getting some much-needed rest at the moment—should I disturb him?" A secretary can say smilingly, "I do hope you two won't get to visiting, because we're behind schedule this afternoon."

What about the frustrating patients who fail to follow directions—particularly the ones who don't stick to a reducing diet or who refuse to give up smoking or alcohol? Antagonism between patient and doctor may be especially marked if the doctor himself is a "reformed sinner" in the field. The difficulty comes when we assume that others can give up pleasures as easily as we. "If I can do it, you can" is a statement devoid of empathy and almost always odious. How is one to measure the pleasure another gets from a given act or the pain he experiences from withdrawal? Besides, most physicians are emotionally more mature than most patients, and self-denial requires maturity.

The physician who rejects patients for failure to follow directions risks pushing them to those who will ask less of them or to those who will offer quick, quack cures or dangerous substitutes. This is not to say that good therapy must condone intemperance or failure to cooperate. The chapter on motivating patients discusses this problem more fully.

An occasional patient will test me by indicating that he has failed to take the medicine I prescribed for him. Here I say, "Why do you pay good money for my services when you don't accept my treatment?" If a reasonable answer is not forthcoming it may be assumed that this patient is playing games. If confrontation doesn't work, I may throw in my hand with a fairly clear conscience.

Others who don't take their medicine express fear of the medication or complain of bizarre side effects. These are often depressed people who don't believe anything can help them, who don't want to be better, or who have fears of losing their minds or self-control under the influence of "drugs," as they refer to medication.

Depression is one of the commonest diseases. When unrecognized, it can cause illness and suffering that persist for years—and it can produce some most difficult problem patients. Almost never does a patient say, "I'm blue" or, "I'm depressed" or, "I'm down in the dumps," but he'll readily admit to these feelings if the doctor expresses them for him. Listen for the solitary, sighing respiration; so far as I know, this common and characteristic deep breath is pathognomonic of depression. Dr. Walter Alvarez described it as a cardinal sign of "caught-in-a-trap disease." If frequent and uncontrolled, these sighs go on to symptoms of hyperventilation—giddiness, paresthesias, headaches, semicoma ("blackout spells")—and are associated with chest tightening and globus.

Depressed people usually admit (on direct questioning only)

to early-morning insomnia, tearfulness ("I could cry if anyone just looks at me"), circular, repetitious thinking ("I'm afraid I'm losing my mind"), feelings of uselessness, inability to love themselves or others, and hopelessness. They are commonly convinced that no one can possibly understand or help them. In severe cases suicide is possible, so they should always be asked directly, "Have you been so depressed that you've thought of doing away with yourself?"

It may be very difficult to convince these people that help is at hand. And because depression can be contagious, the therapist may have to fight an impulse to get away. Then there's the discomfort that female tears arouse in the male breast.

Certainly the Pollyanna approach of "Cheer up, everything's going to be all right" only further isolates these unhappy people, while sympathy stimulates new freshets of tears. My approach is to convince the patient that I know how he feels, by describing symptoms to him that he hasn't told me about. Then I try to convince him that depression is a very real disease and that it can be treated. Next I prescribe one of the psychic energizers, discuss possible side effects, and make him promise to call me before he discontinues medication. If possible, it's good to have a relative in at this time to ensure that the prescription will be purchased and taken. Finally, I assure the patient of my personal concern and involvement by setting another appointment in the near future, no more than a week or two away. I often call the most severely depressed or lonely people by telephone every few days, ostensibly to check on progress, but actually to give them a feeling that someone cares; one thing depressed people usually respond to is T.L.C. Thanks to that and our new drugs, it doesn't take long to see improvement in most cases.

By contrast with these weak, defeated problem patients, there's the irate, chip-on-the-shoulder, "Why-don't-you-doctors-make-house-calls?" individual, who tests one's saintliness severely. Penetrate the outer crust and you will often discover a frightened, love-starved human being, fending off people whom he fears. He fears people who threaten his security by trying to penetrate him—to become intimate with him—for fear that they might then abandon, dominate, or demand too much of him. An insecure doctor may bristle back, and the two will part, each fortified in his belief that one must always keep his guard up.

The secure physician, on the other hand, confident that all people are basically alike in hunger for friendship, will ignore the crust and ask himself, "What is this man afraid of?" The answer will usually be that he fears those he depends on will abandon him, as has happened to him in the past. So he is testing the doctor's mettle—his ability to stand up under fire—to be sure he can be trusted.

The understanding physician then sees him as a particular challenge. If successful, the doctor will probably attract a whole practice of cantankerous curmudgeons, for these, of all patients, must drift and search long among us to find an understanding and trustworthy tamer. One of the most useful approaches to these people is that of bantering humor. It's difficult to fear a person relaxed enough to crack jokes, and one can trust a person confident enough to meet anger with banter. The exchange might go something like this:

NEW PATIENT: I don't know why I'm wasting your time. Doctors aren't able to find out what's wrong with me. I wish we had the old-fashioned doctors we used to have.

SMILING DOCTOR: So long as you pay your bills, my time isn't wasted, but *you* may be wasting your money. Anyway, I'll try to be as old-fashioned as possible.

If the subject responds with a gleam, the approach is keyed right, and the relationship is off to a respectful start. Depressed patients, however, will resent good spirits in a doctor and respond negatively to this approach. For them, warmth and empathy are more effective, as for example when the Mona-Lisa-smiling doctor says: "I'm sorry you've had so much trouble finding an answer to your problems. Tell me what it was you liked most about the old-fashioned doctor."

In neither instance has the physician risen to the proffered bait and defended modern doctors against the old-fashioned variety. To do so would start a "win-lose" argument in which each participant might well reject the other.

Finally, it's customary to talk of the patient who threatens to become *too* intimate: a danger, like that of having too much money, which may be more theoretical than real. It's doubtful that any physician who is mature and self-approving encounters problems with seductive patients. But physicians who fear close personal relationships may see seduction lurking behind every personal remark their patients make, and some physicians may semiconsciously encourage sexual advances.

In any event, my aides usually tip me off; as women, they're quick to spot brazen caprice. They usually take a dislike to such a patient and may drive her off with dark looks, acid responses, and delayed appointments. Failing that, they may amaze me by expressing their dislike; to this point, I will have thought of the relationship as merely pleasant and attractive.

The solution is not to throw the patient out (unless the physician fears he can't withstand her siren call, in which case *he* should see a psychiatrist), but rather to damp the flames of passion. Since this is largely a treatise on the production of *more* intimacy with patients, one might simply turn the book upside down and read it backwards to learn how to cool off doctor-patient relations. Fortunately, few of us need to be schooled in how to turn people off; somewhere along the line we have almost certainly been taught *that* art by masters.

In the case of the seductive female, a "professionally correct" manner should be sufficiently chilling. If not, some indication that the doctor is happily married to "The Most Wonderful Woman in the World" (the antithesis of "My wife doesn't really understand me") should do the job.

That brings us to the unhappy subject of how to reject patients. This chapter started with the admission that we all have some people we simply can't stand. Usually this will be so apparent that prompt separation occurs. Still, a few masochists will come back for more. There are some patients (and perhaps a few doctors) who can only form comfortable relationships in a milieu of hostility; hate is so much more dependable than love, and so much easier to engender. The role-playing physician who tries to please everybody may perforate his ulcer or send himself to Lexington over small proportion of misfits when it is far easier and, in the long run, kinder to send them packing.

Before that, it's wise to make an attempt to rehabilitate the relationship—like this: "John, I'm having trouble with you. My experience tells me that when I find it hard to get along with a patient it's because of some fault on both sides. Perhaps if you tell me how I rub you wrong I'll be a better doctor for it. Frankly, you upset me by . . ."

Naturally, such a direct confrontation requires utmost tact. No matter what the patient says, the physician must thank him, promise to do better, and keep a warm smile on his face. The doctor need not agree, but he should listen very carefully because the chances are that other patients have the same objections. It takes courage and maturity to walk up to a true mirror and take a long, hard look. Most people live out their lives without daring to inquire—with a sincere desire for an honest answer —about their faults.

Still we all have our limitations. When all else fails, it is wrong to retain a patient one hates: bad for him, bad for the doctor, and bad for the profession. Getting out of such a relationship may be more difficult for an insecure doctor than getting into one. The techniques for doing so are described in Chapter 18.

It's common in obstetrics to have on the wall a framed question: "Is this an ectopic?" As a final note on problem patients I'd like to propose that each angry, frustrated, rejecting physician bring himself up short in the same way by asking, "Why isn't this patient a schizophrenic?" It's extraordinary how much more I can tolerate from a patient once I've labeled him schizophrenic. To paraphrase an oldtime comedian, "Difficult patients are the craziest people!"

CHAPTER 12

Ways to Deal With Chronics

Sometimes I think the hotshot diagnostician and the big-shot surgeon have the easiest jobs in medicine: They tear into a case with a definite goal in mind and take off while the applause is still ringing.

The real hero in medicine, it sometimes seems to me, is the guy that takes care of patients who never recover completely, rarely improve, and usually deteriorate, at a snail's pace. Looking back, I don't think anyone prepared me as a student for the fact that I'd be seeing the same diabetics, hypertensives, arthritics, and cardiacs for years and years and years, knowing that we were always fighting a futile battle.

I can still remember the bitterness of a few years back when I achieved the temporary triumph of getting one of my hypertensive-stroke patients titered to a proper proportion of pills so he could endure a long-postponed trip to Florida—on which he was smashed dead in an auto accident. He'd probably be alive today, safe in some local nursing home, if I hadn't taken such careful care of him.

There are some special hazards in the field that merit discussion: First, of course, is the monotony. Once a diagnosis is made and treatment has been initiated, the pace of a case slows to such crucial decisions as whether to prescribe one pill or two, to be taken before meals or after. The monotony is enlivened only by emergency calls asking what to do if a dose is skipped and whether it's safe to take aspirin at the same time.

Boredom is not only unpleasant for me, but when my patient senses it (as he will) he'll be doubly hurt by a hopeless disease and an unenthusiastic doctor. And I imagine my patients get a little bored, too, having the same questions and tests followed by the same injunctions at every visit.

Then there's the risk of prejudice. After we look at a thing repeatedly we stop seeing it. (That's why we don't notice the little woman's new hairdo.) I remember a diabetic who came to the office so often that I stopped looking at him until his wife asked about his pallor—which taught me that diabetics get cancers in their colons, too. If he'd been a new patient that day I'd have noticed his anemia when he walked in the door. And we develop a prejudiced feeling that all of our neurotics' symptoms are functional in origin—certainly you can supply your own horrible examples of that.

There's the difficulty of deciding how often a patient should return. Nobody has fed the computer digestible facts to tell us the optimum interval between visits. Somehow, the OB men have determined how often it's best to see pregnant ladies, but I think that's more a reflection of their love of routine than a product of scientific calculation. For post-coronary patients, ulcer patients, people with glaucoma, and many others there are no guidelines. When the Michigan Society of Internal Medicine surveyed its members a while back about how often a man aged

80 should have a physical exam, they got answers that ranged all the way from "monthly" to "never." Somehow the decision is made by each doctor, according to his training and nature, on the basis of his understanding of both his patient's willingness to pay and his need of reassurance, plus their mutual anxiety over the seriousness of the disease. There's danger of overcompensation in scheduling return visits, too. In the early days of practice a doctor may see his patients *less* often than he should because he's afraid of being motivated by his need for more business. Later on, he may see them *too* often because he's afraid he'll be accused of being too busy to take care of people as well as he should.

There's frustration in not being able to bring people all the miracles modern medicine is supposed to offer and in trying to explain why, in a technology that's wiping out polio, we still don't know what causes acne and vitiligo and psoriasis. Since most of us went into medicine to cure people, it's downright disheartening to tot up the diseases we treat but never cure.

Still, although the hotshots might not agree, there are some rewards and challenges in taking care of chronics. It's a matter of the doctor's temperament, I suppose, to be able to enjoy seeing the same people with the same diseases and the same complaints again and again. Some people read a book once and are done with it, while others reread their favorites many times.

Anyway, it has to be done. Here are some precepts that help me in dealing with the chronic:

To fend off boredom, I try to mix it up a little by making each visit a fresh approach. For a hypertensive I might take the blood pressure in both arms on some occasions, and after rest or exercise on others. I try to spend a little time talking about some nonmedical subject of interest to him, and I've tried to keep from harping too often on the theme of "take-off-weight-and-stop-smoking." (A patient once told me that I *always* brought that subject up, and he was tired of it.) I can still see the astonished look on the face of one of my emphysema patients when I checked him over and didn't once inquire (as had been my routine for years) whether he'd stopped smoking yet. It was hard but worthwhile, because he then saw that while taking care of the emphysema was *my* job, the smoking was *his*. Once in a while the monotony can be relieved by trying a new medicine, discovering that it doesn't work, and returning to the former regimen.

To help determine the interval until the next visit, I'd suggest watching for clues from the patient as to what *he* expects. Often he'll register some complaint about cost to indicate he thinks he's coming too often. If he expresses some apprehension about his disease, on the other hand, it may indicate that he needs reassurance more frequently. It's wise to be careful about changing the frequency of visits. If they're stepped up it's sure to suggest that his condition is worse; if they're cut down he may assume that you're trying to slough his problem. And I think it's important to charge enough for return visits so that they don't become "loss leaders." Admit it or not, money is a powerful subconscious motivator for doctors. If a man's gross is $30 an hour and he likes to spend 20 minutes on each of a diabetic's visits, then the proper charge is $10. Anything less and there's danger he'll subconsciously either lengthen the interval between visits, shorten the time he spends on each visit, or begin to find the treatment of diabetics dreary.

The chronic's doctor must lay hands on the affected part *each time*. Woe unto me if I see a hypertensive and forget to take the blood pressure, or dismiss a spastic colon without prodding the belly. Peculiarly, my patients seldom mention such omissions at the time, when I'd have a chance to recoup; they wait until the next visit and *then* spring the trap: "How come you didn't ask for a specimen last time, like you always do?"

To avoid diagnostic complacency I try to make sure that each of my chronics gets a thorough checkup once a year. If it's important for healthy people to have regular examinations, it's doubly so for the handicapped. On those occasions I try to forget the primary disease and go looking for all the complications and other diseases I can find. Lightning *does* strike twice in the same place, as indicated by a 35-year-old lady in my practice who has myxedema, diabetes, vitiligo, *and* multiple sclerosis.

It's only fair to the chronic, and it improves cooperation, to warn him at the onset about what he's getting into in terms of visits and expense. To a new diabetic my instruction includes a statement like this:

"There isn't any cure for your disease, so your welfare depends on our working closely together to keep you in the best possible shape. Until we get your sugar controlled I'll see you every week or two and call on the telephone between visits. Later it won't be necessary for you to come so often, but for the present I'd like you to come in for a check on your blood sugar at least every three months, and we require a complete physical examination yearly. We'll be responsible for keeping track of your appointments and call you when it's time to come in, but if we slip up anytime and you realize you haven't seen us in over three months, please jog us. What with your medicine, you'd better figure on medical expenses of $100 to $200 a year.

"Oh yes, and be sure to keep up your hospitalization insurance. Diabetics use hospitals about twice as much as other people because even a little illness can throw a diabetic's control out of kilter and land him in the hospital for a few days."

Any intelligent person with a chronic disease goes right to the library as soon as he hears the diagnosis. There's nothing we can do to stop him, and there's some advantage in his learning all he can—after all, it's his disease. The problem is that he's going to read about all the complications and life expectancy of atypical cases, which will depress him until he can build up some denial defenses. During that depressed period he'll be barred from access to my reassurance by his embarrassment over having gone to the books without telling me.

The best solution I've found is to give him all the reading material I can in the form of pamphlets put out by the voluntary health agencies. These are always written in a reassuring manner, and they never, never bring up such unpleasant subjects as death. And then I *urge* him to go to the library and even suggest some source materials he can ask for there. But to be more sure he *won't* go (in case my suggesting it is not a strong enough deterrent), I add, "You'll find a lot of big scientific terms you won't understand, and they may scare you, so don't hesitate to call me and I'll interpret them for you."

After that, there'll be the problem of all those well-intentioned friends and relatives—damn their eyes—who give him case histories of the people they know who've died horribly, or worse yet, achieved a complete cure, and why doesn't he ask his doctor about it? And, just about then, there's bound to be a long article in the news media about some "new hope" for victims of his disease, based on something a junior scientist has observed in ferrets that might be tried on humans if he can reproduce the results in guinea pigs.

Here too, I try to get in the first blow by saying, "Your friends are going to be anxious to help you by sending you clippings and reports of other treatments for your trouble. Get all the information you can for me, bring it in when you come, and, if it looks promising, we'll try it out on you and see if it works. If it does, and there are no *severe* side effects, I'll use it on my other patients, too." It's funny, but offhand I can't remember when anyone's taken me up on that offer.

Unusual and serious chronic disease—such as chronic leukemia, multiple sclerosis, and lupus—will usually prompt some friend or relative to suggest to the patient that he ought to be seen in some university clinic or big medical center. That's pretty good advice—if I had one of those conditions I'd want to go to the top, too. So, as I get older and wiser, I send them off right at the outset and work with the patient and the medical center from then on. Before I learned my lesson, I'd have the patient for a few months, then he'd go elsewhere on his own and be too embarrassed to come back.

Finally, as an ex-victim of a chronic disease myself, let me make a plea for being absolutely honest with the patient and his relatives from the start. Resist that impulse to soften the blow by painting a rosier future than the situation warrants. If it's going to be a two-year or a lifetime proposition, say so. There are few situations more frightening than being treated for a serious disease by a doctor who sometimes keeps things from you.

One thing about the chronics, they get to be old personal friends—almost members of the office family. We don't have to keep up a front with them, and it's hard to imagine they'd ever spark one of those malpractice suits that big-shot surgeons live in fear of. Spaced through the day, their visits can be as relaxing as coffee breaks.

They can even be inspiring. Having an incurable illness puts a person's back against the wall. It can bring out the worst in him, but in most it's the best that shows through. I guess we all have a few patients whose cheerful courage in the face of pain and disability brightens the whole office for hours after they leave.

Patients to
nstructions

I well remember my ... n the early days of practice when I tried to induce my patients to follow given courses of action and found that most of them simply wouldn't.

As a result *I* suffered: a sense of impotence at being unable to impose my judgments on them, feelings of personal failure, rage at being hoodwinked, sorrow that they were denying themselves the benefits I knew cooperation could bring them, and self-recrimination for not having approached them correctly. That's quite a basket of emotions for a young man with wet ears.

In medical school I was taught that the first step in treating diabetics and hypertensives is to reduce them to ideal weight, so when I started practice I waded into all my overindulging patients. It wasn't until I'd been in practice a whole month that I discovered my clientele could be sorted into three bins:

1. A few who already had excellent habits.
2. A few who were thick-skinned and masochistic enough to put up with my lectures but who continued to transgress.
3. The many who took their bad habits to less zealous doctors.

The fourth category, those who followed advice, existed only in the minds of those remote enough from the practice of medicine to teach it. That left me specializing in the healthy first group and the obdurate second group, when the third was where the action lay.

I went through a period of nihilistic indifference—and practice picked up. Then came a phase in which I tried pills—appetite suppressants, tranquilizers, vitamin placebos—that gave me and the patient a feeling something was being done. But if any benefit resulted, it ceased when the dose was cut. Sometimes the patient became addicted to the pills, replacing one bad habit with a worse one.

My feelings of frustration about overindulging, health-neglecting patients haven't been completely resolved, but I've transferred some of my rage to the boys in the ivory towers who have spent millions on medical research and almost nothing on motivational research. What good does it do to discover that weight loss promotes health if we don't discover how to motivate people to diet and exercise? We've known for a long time that a third of the pills we prescribe aren't taken, but we do nothing about developing techniques to improve the situation.

Look at coronary artery disease: It's the largest single cause of death in this country, yet most of it is preventable. "All" we have to do is get every man, woman, and child to avoid cigarettes, keep thin, and run two miles a day. That's a pretty tough challenge, but it's not impossible, as evidenced by the fact that a third of our own profession have given up cigarettes. Yet we're able to induce less than 10 per cent of the population to follow our example.

I think we share the blame for this curious breach in our armament against disease. First, the patient's breach is the doctor's shield; patient noncooperation is our most frequent excuse for our own failures. If everyone did exactly as we said, we'd *have* to produce better results.

Second, the people in clinics and medical schools often lack the intimate, prolonged contact with patients that we who are in practice have. They may see a fat lady initially, refer her to a dietitian for instructions, and never see her again to learn how futile it is to treat obesity solely with diets.

And third, I think we find it undignified and demeaning to "sell"; we prefer "doctor's orders." Yet selling is what motivation is all about. Actually, most of our work is in the entirely uncharted realm of "anti-selling" or *de*-motivation. It's one thing to sell an Eskimo a refrigerator and quite another to sell his fat wife on keeping her nose out of it. A lot of what we try to sell involves self-denial rather than self-indulgence. In the whole field of commerce, the only people whose occupational difficulty approaches ours are those who try to induce people to *save* money (insurance salesmen, bankers) rather than spend it.

And, finally, we're denied the salesman's aid of impulse buying, because giving up smoking, overeating, and alcohol require *lifelong* self-denial of pleasures that were once highly satisfying.

So let's look at some of the factors that move people to change —to deny rather than indulge. Again, we're dealing in contracts, so it will be important to consider what the patient is to give and what he's to get. Unless that concept is clear, the cause is almost certainly doomed. A peremptory order to carry out an act because it's demanded by the authority figure may work in military life, but it's almost certain to have the opposite effect on intelligent civilians.

Most doctors, I'm afraid, use the mature approach of appealing to reason. That may be direct, simple, logical, and effective if the task required is simple, or the patient is suffering. "Take one of these every four hours for pain" is an injunction that requires only a little sacrifice (swallowing a pill) for a larger and, hopefully, immediate reward (relief of pain).

But the logical approach won't work nearly so well when the balance involves more sacrifice—"Lift this weight 30 times with each foot to strengthen your quadriceps muscle"—or less reward, as represented by the frequency with which people forget medicine prescribed for asymptomatic conditions such as diabetes or hypertension. In any event, the mature approach requires mature patients, and they're rare, especially in the fields of alcoholism and obesity; immaturity is always a cardinal feature of those diseases.

So the next approach many of us try is to create *anxiety*. I notice that almost every doctor we ask to speak to our alcoholic groups starts out talking about cirrhosis of the liver, pancreatitis, and Korsakoff's brain damage.

Fear is a potent motivator for a short time, but it's limited as a long-term motivator unless it's supported by reality. A man who is feeling the pain of a coronary knows reality, and an injunction to stop smoking given at that point will usually work. As we've all observed, it's much easier to motivate the patient who already has a disease than the one who's being urged to avoid it. Immature and insecure people find it easy to believe that the disease we're warning against will hit the other guy, but not them. That's why 90 per cent of the population can believe that smoking is bad for health, yet keep consuming cigarettes at the same rate.

If you want to move a donkey, we're told, you should hit him with a stick and dangle a carrot before his snout. People, too, move away from pain and toward pleasure. But carrots, like fear, spoil over the long course. Sooner or (usually) later, the pain of the disease will force patient compliance, but usually by then it's tragically too late.

Guilt is a powerful motivator for the alcoholic, the compulsive gambler, and the housewife with a tranquilizer-sleeping pill problem, but I'm not sure we, as doctors, are prepared to shame people into change. Somehow it doesn't seem like a good, clean weapon in our hands, and even preachers and judges don't use it as much as they once did.

Money should be a motivator. I once tried seeing weight-reduction patients for nothing, to encourage them to come in. Then I tried charging double for visits when they'd failed to lose and nothing when they had. But neither scheme seemed to make much difference in the patient—though the second approach of course did something for my income. For years I couldn't think of any other potions in the doctor's motivational pharmacopoeia.

But there were scattered patients who roiled my complacency by reforming at the hands of other agencies. How was it that an evangelist could give a hard-core reprobate enough religion in one short sermon to cure him of wine, women, and tobacco for life? Why could Alcoholics Anonymous claim 50 per cent success rate with alcoholics when psychiatrists admitted to less than 10 per cent? What motivated those who gave up their self-destructive habits spontaneously?

I can't claim to have all the answers yet, but contact with thousands of alcoholics has taught me some principles that seem to be transferable to all the compulsions and "diseases of overindulgence." (Victims of food, cigarettes, and alcohol head the list of sufferers, but it includes drug and narcotic addicts, hypochondriacs, compulsive workers and gamblers, masochists with a compulsion to be operated upon or to marry men who will beat them, and even those Carry Nation-like zealots who are addicted to fighting addictions.)

The closest approach to the proper application of the principles can be observed in the work of the evangelist, the football coach, or the Marine drill sergeant. They, too, work with immature personalities, and they succeed through leadership in establishing an esprit among members of a group who are held together by identification with each other, fear of rejection by peers, and enthusiasm for the group and its leader.

Applied to medical practice, this means that our traditional relationships with our clientele can seldom do the trick. An occasional victim will mature out of his problem by himself, but the rest will have to continue to suffer with little help from us —unless we change our approach and encourage or initiate group therapy for our patients.

If necessary, we can lead the groups ourselves; it doesn't take much training. There's no reason why one doctor can't preach to a congregation of fatties while another coaches a team of smokers and a third drills a platoon of alcoholics. At the very least we can encourage our patients to prolonged participation in A.A., T.O.P.S. (Take Off Pounds Sensibly), Weight Watchers, Inc., Gamblers Anonymous, Recovery, Inc. (for compulsive hypochondriacs), Synanon (narcotic addiction), and The Seven Step Foundation (for habitual criminals). At the most, we can set up classes for dietary treatment of diabetic and cardiac patients and clinics for smoking withdrawal and alcoholism—all of which are now in operation in the general hospital where I practice. They could be initiated as readily by any medium-sized clinic or group. I know of one doctor who ran classes for alcoholics in an old house converted for this purpose.

Why do these self-help groups have such a high rate of success? The explanation lies largely in those words "self-help" and "group."

One motivator we've almost never used is to *make the patient a doctor to others with his own problem.* Being doctors has forced a third of *us* to stop smoking. Give a smoker the job of helping others to quit, and he'll have to set (and keep) an example. As a means of helping everyone equally, almost all of these groups have very little leadership, and that little is changed frequently to give everyone a chance to be "doctor." In the best-run groups, everyone treats everybody.

The next most important secret of the groups' success is that they mobilize *peer pressure*. Most people *start* smoking or drinking because it's "the thing to do" in the peer group they belong to or aspire to join; they're afraid they'll be rejected as squares if they don't go along with the group. They can *stop* drinking and smoking through the same kind of influence. When an alcoholic goes to A.A. he leaves a group that approves of getting drunk and joins one that strongly disapproves of drinking and favors staying sober. Most advertising of such things as automobiles and clothes and cigarettes is designed to create just such pressures of peer-group opinion. When we can make cigarette-smoking unfashionable, cigarettes will cease to be a problem. We've already been fairly successful in creating a peer acceptance of thinness. Who ever saw a fat fashion model?

Furthermore, groups sustain effort by meeting frequently (sometimes every night in the week), by surrounding the transgressor with the reality of fellow sinners who didn't stop in time or who "fell off the wagon," and by keeping the member's interest high for a long period of time. Originally, the neophyte goes *for* help, but shortly he becomes enthusiastic about going *to* help. When that occurs he's almost always hooked.

The groups for fatties have the toughest job because they can only counsel moderation while the others can preach abstinence. As any ex-smoker can tell you, it's much easier to cut out than to cut down. But that very handicap gives weight reducers the motivational advantage of *competition*. In a way, alcoholics compete to see who can stay sober the longest, but they're not in the same league with a couple of ladies racing each other to get down to 150 pounds for the prize of a 400-calorie dinner out.

In the end, groups accomplish the same deeper goals we

doctors have—to help people mature, to give them insight, to make them more relaxed, happier, and "well adjusted"—because a group, no matter what its composition, is inherently psycho-therapeutic.

Nowadays when compulsive patients show up I'm no longer frustrated. I say something like this: "Mrs. Jones, like many others, you have a bad habit that is already affecting your health." (Motivation is much stronger when the damage is already apparent than when it is still theoretical.) "You must stop immediately, and *for the rest of your life.*" (This is important: Once an individual has achieved an excessive level of any pleasure-giving substance or activity he can almost never stop and come back to satisfaction at any lower dose. Except for the dieter, immediate total and lifelong abstinence is best, and even the dieter must diet the rest of his life—not just for 18 days.)

"This is hard to do," I continue, "but not impossible, and it gets easier. Fortunately, we have a group of people in the same boat who will help you. One of the important benefits of this group is that shortly you will be helping others, which will strengthen your resolution and keep you from relapsing."

At this point, the usual patient will have only the faintest desire to comply, so it's time to apply the hammerlock: "I'm going to call one of my patients who is active in this work and have her pick you up and take you to the first meeting. Someday I'll be calling on you to do the same for someone else." And right then and there I make the call and the appointment, trying to match my patient with someone of similar background from her own part of town.

Short of flat refusal or breaking a leg, there is no way she can escape that first meeting. Once there, the chances are she will continue. One evangelist can be pretty persuasive; a roomful can overpower the strongest sinner. The leaven of the group will not begin to froth, though, until my patient converts her first cohort.

From then on she'll be an enthusiast and, having led one convert to the altar, she'll be much less likely to backslide herself.

But I won't abandon her to the group abruptly: I'll continue to see her at intervals for many months to give encouragement. In the average case, even after two years of unbroken success, there remains a 20 per cent chance of backsliding. Particularly dangerous is the three-month point when desire for what's forbidden has faded. Then it will be easy for her to believe she no longer needs the group. If she stops going she will next decide that it's safe to indulge a little, since she no longer has a craving. If she does, she'll be back at her former dose within a few weeks.

Does this mean that we must always get a patient into a group if we are to help him? Of course not. Even if that *were* true, many doctors practice in areas where groups are not operating. But I think, where they are available, groups provide the most effective means of helping patients with these tough problems.

For day-to-day patient motivation here are discussions of some principles that I think will help:

The best help arises out of a close personal relationship, or, put another way, a good salesman sells himself as well as his product. Before our patients trust our advice they'll have to believe in us. Without imitating the charlatan's duplicity, we can learn from his success at selling some remarkably crude devices and remedies by overwhelming his clients with "personality" and projecting an image of honesty and sincerity. As we've said repeatedly in this book, the closer the doctor-patient relationship, the more productive of desired change it's apt to be.

Behind every refusal to cooperate there's a reason. People are not often too stupid to follow orders, nor do they fail to change because they like to see us unhappy. If they don't follow the advice they've requested and are paying for it's usually because they're "hung up" on some barrier to change. Discover and remove that barrier, and the problem may move much closer to solution. So I always approach the recalcitrant patient saying to myself: "If this person saw the world as I do and knew what I know, he'd do as I do—now, what's the difference between us?" Sometimes the difference is that I have more knowledge than he; sometimes it's a matter of prejudice or phobia. ("I don't like to take medicine" or, "If I don't have pills I won't sleep a wink.") More often it's fear and innate resistance to change, buttressed by a well-polished alibi system that must be broken down. But *be gentle.* When you start pulling down a man's protective walls his roof can fall in, too.

In overcoming rationalizations, excuses, and alibis, I find it's best to avoid sarcasm and direction contradictions, because they belittle the patient and make him struggle harder to resist me. Much safer is the adroit question that impales him on his own illogic. There *has* to be a cardinal fault in every alibi because the alibi leads to the conclusion that the act is right when, in fact, it is wrong. If that fault can be shown to the patient he will no longer be able to use that particular alibi—he may go on to others but in time he'll run out of excuses and will have to face the reality of his situation. For example, say an alcoholic rationalizes that he drinks a lot of martinis just because he likes the flavor. An excellent response is, "Would you pay a dollar for a small glass of clear liquid that tasted just the same, but had no alcohol in it?"

A frequent parry against giving up "comfort-producing chemicals" (to use Dr. Gordon Bell's phrase) is the retort, "I can stop if I want to; I did it once." To which I answer, "I'm afraid that was only a 'vacation.' You couldn't have quit, because you're back at it now. I'm suggesting that you quit absolutely, permanently, and forever, which is quite different from anything you've done before."

Sometimes tasks can be set that confront the patient with reality. The fat lady who "eats like a bird" can be requested to keep a diary of every mouthful she eats for a few days; the person who says he lights a lot of cigarettes but doesn't smoke them down should be asked to have his wife collect the butts from his ash trays and send them in for measurement. And, again, exposure of the alibier to his peers will puncture his defenses. The doctor's not in a position to laugh at him but *they* are, and will, uproariously.

In prescribing diets, medicines, or treatments that are onerous we could learn from the auto industry to tailor our product to the customer's tastes. We've had help from the pharmaceutical manufacturers who've discovered, for example, that people are more likely to take cough syrup if it's red. If a neurotic "can't" swallow pills, I give him everything in liquid form. A diet that fails to consider strong distastes or religious requirements simply won't work; if I can't work out a compromise I call in a dietitian.

Flexibility helps. My children have taught me that rigidity begets rigidity. For example, if I tell my youngsters to "stop that right now" or "go to bed this instant" there's resistance. But if I say, "You can do that only five more times" or, "Bedtime in ten minutes" it gives them a chance to display some autonomy.

I think we could do a better job of confronting patients with reality than we sometimes do. When a salesman says, "Those tires have 20,000 miles on them," it doesn't move me much, but when the grease monkey shows me a spot where the tread is gone he makes a sale right then. So when I hear wheezes in a smoker, I put the stethoscope on him and let *him* hear them. I make alcoholics feel their own liver edge and show them spider nevi and liver palms. Even when fat ladies come solely for the relief of symptoms of a common cold they get weighed—it's not surprising that many of them never step on the scales at home.

In motivating people to accept elective surgery, it's wise to give the patient a "choice." Better than issuing a direct order—"You've got to have an operation"—is the technique of sharing our knowledge with him and letting him feel *he*'s made the decision. I may say, for example: "I can usually bring you through these attacks, but sooner or later there'll be one when I can't, and then you'll need emergency surgery, possibly when it's least convenient. Sooner or later it's going to have to come out— I never knew of a case that got better by itself—but you can suit yourself as to whether you want it done now."

Sometimes motivation is enhanced by getting the family into the act, but it has to be done right; nagging makes things worse, and I certainly wouldn't want to set a wife up as her husband's keeper. However, I've found that reducing diets work better when two members of a household participate; similarly a man is more apt to stop smoking if his wife joins him in the effort. That way, each member hesitates to transgress for fear he'll take the other's resolution down the drain with him.

A high rate of relapse is to be expected in the early stages of breaking bad habits. Most smokers "stop" several times before they make it. Someone once said, "There's no such thing as an 18-day diet or even a 5-day diet—there's only a *one*-day diet. After that, everybody starts cheating." The important things to observe in handling relapses are: Don't get your feelings hurt if shame makes the patient fib a little; don't get angry, or he'll never come back; don't condone the relapse but do use it productively to show him that he's up against a lifelong problem for which there is no easy or temporary solution. And try to help him discover the triggers and attitudes that set off his fall from grace, so he'll be on guard the next time similar circumstances arise. If he's been in a group, he'll almost always have left the group weeks before it happened, so get him back and try to keep him back. Two years of involvement and total and unrelenting abstinence are average requirements before there's a reasonable chance of success in most of these conditions. Accordingly, it's best if he doesn't get his rewards too fast. If, on his first return visit, I praise an ex-smoker and tell him how much clearer his lungs are, he's apt to relapse with the notion that he can undo the effects of his habit in a hurry any time he wants to. I find it's best to sustain and protract his anxiety for as long as possible, while still giving him praise and encouragement.

If relapses are chronic you're probably the unwitting victim of a "game" played by a patient who enjoys being chased, lectured, and rescued—one who is trying to reap alternately the rewards of sin and virtue. At *that* point, stern confrontation and temporary rejection can be tried. You may lose the patient (in which event you'll be spared the frustration of the hopeless cases that are an inevitable segment of the compulsive diseases). But try to leave the door open so he'll be able to crawl back when his habit precipitates a crisis in his life. Even when you fail *before* their heart attacks to convince your patients that they should stop smoking, you can almost always do so immediately after an attack.

That brings up another principle: Strike while the pain is hot. Motivation comes in impulses. If an alcoholic calls for rescue at 11 P.M., members of A.A. respond immediately. An appointment even as early as the following morning will usually be broken. As soon as I'm sure of the diagnosis of myocardial infarction, I tell the victim he's going to stop smoking and get gaunt. At that point he's delighted to hear it because it gives him a positive action program for avoiding further pain.

It's foolish to expect 100 per cent success; 50 per cent is more realistic. But that's better than our batting average with many other diseases. In the case of fat adolescent girls or alcoholics, even 5 per cent might be worth the effort.

As Hippocrates said, "Drastic diseases merit drastic therapy." One of our problems in these conditions is that we often act as though we think obesity, smoking, and alcoholism really *aren't* serious. At least in the case of alcoholism, we can motivate almost every victim to try to stop—if we're really resolute. How? By getting him fired, divorced, or committed to a state hospital. It's tragic to contemplate that almost every cirrhotic skid-row character that I encounter could have been salvaged at some time if someone had only cared enough to use a drastic remedy. Many employers are now using threatened loss of job as a powerful motivator for alcoholic employes, with success rates as high as 80 per cent. The Armed Forces have occasionally cracked down on overweight officers and noncoms. So far as I know, no corporation has yet done anything about smoking, but I wonder why not when I contemplate what it must cost to replace top executives dying of coronaries and lung cancer.

I suspect a lot of our problem in motivating patients rests in our own failure to perceive reality; our own beliefs that some magic will spare our patient; our own failure to care enough to do our very best; our own failure to explore techniques long known to the business world.

One more thing, before you tell other people how to behave. I hope that you practice moderation in all things and at all times. It's very hard for a fat doctor to get good results in the treatment of obesity, and an alcoholic doctor seems to fail in the treatment of almost everything.

CHAPTER 14

Relations With Patients' Relations

Recently some of the people who believe that roses will smell sweeter if called by other names have embarked on the task of changing "General Practice" to "Family Practice"—as though all other doctors treated isolated orphans, bachelors, and old maids. Surely, everyone learns at his psychiatry professor's knee of family interactions: that a family is a basic dynamic unit in society; a gear box of toothed personalities meshing with or mashing each other; transmitting or absorbing power, attenuated by noisy friction, lubricated by love.

How presumptuous to believe that any doctor can remachine one gear in that box without considering the alignment of the others! A pediatrician's productivity is entirely proportionate to his parent popularity; obstetricians have classes for expectant fathers; surgeons have special waiting rooms for the relatives of those they're operating upon. One expert in the unhappy field of malpractice has stated that he has never known a suit to be filed if the move was opposed by a single close relative.

Treat the whole family? Who can afford not to? The art is to enlist them in aiding our efforts, or, if that's not possible, at least to neutralize their opposition.

As we've been taught, in an ideally normal family each adult should be capable of the mature, "giving" sort of love, free of hostility and self-centeredness, and possessed of emotional independence. And the older children should be approaching that status. How much rosier the practice of medicine would be if that were true in every family!

As we all know to the contrary, most families are held together with the baling wire of dependency relationships. The eager doctor who starts cutting that wire without understanding what it's holding together may never get the machine back together again.

So let's discuss some of these dependency relationships, not from the standpoint of what they do to the dominating-submitting patients involved, but from the standpoint of the doctor who is trying to help.

Naturally, dependency doesn't just happen. In children it is instilled by a dominating parent; in marriage it's an attraction of opposites. In either event, where there is dependency there is domination.

Sometimes these "sick" master-slave associations, when they occur between mutually consenting adults, don't threaten my efforts to treat one or the other. Once the relationship is discovered (and *that*'s not hard), I play pediatrician and deal with the dominator as the parent and the dependent as the child.

But at other times one has to free the slaves in order to treat the shackle sores. This can cause civil war, especially when the slaves are afraid of freedom and the mistress can't exist without them—as happens when I try to get a menopausal matron to let her effeminate youngest son become a man.

One of the troublesome dependency relationships in my practice is that of the dominant husband and passive wife in situations where I need a wife's support in motivating the husband, but she's too wishy-washy to stand up to him. In dealing with drug addictions, for example, it's important that the family be enlisted in therapy. If they're too sympathetic when the going gets tough, they may accede to the addict's demands for more medicine (or for a change of doctors) and wreck the whole campaign. One of the most hopeless cases of addiction I've seen in a long time was that of an elderly man whose wife was so dependent on him that she couldn't be parted from him, even for one night. This became apparent when I tried to hospitalize him for withdrawal therapy and she signed him out against advice because I wouldn't let her occupy the adjoining bed. I might have been able to arrange for her to stay, but she would certainly have smuggled drugs to him or taken him out the minute the going got tough.

The moral of this kind of case is: Don't expect a little girl to do a wife's job. You can still treat the dominant husband in the usual case, but you'd better not expect the wife to contribute.

A more commonly troublesome dependency relation is the reverse: the pants-wearing wife and her little-boy husband. Many alcoholic males belong in this category. In these cases the wife, while expressing a desire on a conscious level to be married to a real man, subconsciously resists any threat to her power. (It's dangerous, though, to convict the wife without hearing her version. Every alcoholic would like me to believe that his wife was responsible for scuttling his last period of sobriety, but when I get them together to discuss it, it usually comes out that he fired the first shot, hoping she'd react violently enough to give him an excuse to relapse.)

There *are*, however, a few wives who genuinely need to be married to sick men. No matter how earnestly one of these may proclaim a desire to have her husband well, she'll find fault with any measures that threaten a cure. She's the kind who resists surgery for her husband's hernia or his disk, who can't get the hang of his diabetic diet, or who won't get involved in his medications, dressings, or nursing care. Sometimes she can be spotted because she's sure that medical science has nothing to offer. At other times she'll beg for help with the ailing spouse but then refuse to participate in any program that requires her cooperation.

Whenever I get involved in strong husband-wife conflicts, I try to get the two together and carry on what psychiatrists are now calling "conjoint therapy." (I suspect it's been in existence longer than psychiatrists have, though.) Getting them in my office at the same time, I try to establish in both their minds that I'm eager to be helpful and am sympathetic to both sides without favoring one over the other.

It's easy to see why in the past a psychiatrist usually refused to take on both a husband and wife as his patients. Seeing each partner separately in an attempt to patch up a marriage is about as safe, in my experience, as camping out on a bombing range. When each partner gets back home, he misrepresents half of what was said and, before long, there are three fighters in the ring instead of two. If I'm going to agree with a man that his wife is a scold I want to have her hear it, so she'll also hear me add that if I were his wife, I'm afraid I'd scold, too.

In contrast with the futility of separate treatment, it's astonishing how much good can sometimes be done in a relatively short time with conjoint therapy. Many couples, married for years, are simply unable to communicate with each other. Sometimes, with the help of a sympathetic third person, they can say things (both harsh and tender) they've been holding back for years.

Anyway, the first goal is to get the spouse to see that she is interfering with progress, then to discover why, and next to try to induce her to change. This last is tough because she is often a stubborn, dominating personality who is easily threatened and rigidly protective of the superiority her husband's illness gives her. If all else fails, at least I can show the "man" what he's up against and give him some suggestions for isolating himself.

Should practicing physicians get involved in such marriage counseling? I don't see how a true "family" physician can avoid it. Furthermore, current belief holds that there is rarely such a thing as an isolated case of emotional illness in a family. If Mother is neurotic, a thorough physician will want to understand the kind of man who lives with her. Further, whenever a doctor intervenes effectively to produce a change in the personality of a patient, there's danger he may throw family relationships out of kilter. It's a common experience that when an alcoholic husband achieves sobriety it takes several years before the wife and children learn to live comfortably with the new man in the house.

A milder form of dominating woman is the nagging wife who wants me to speak to her husband about some bad habit—smoking, drinking, and working too hard head the list—but not to mention, of course, that she called. I generally promise to do my best, but warn her that it may not be possible to bring the subject up casually. And then I admonish her about the futility of nagging and try to reassure her that the husband's habit may not be as harmful as she thinks. Chances are she'll never find out whether the matter *was* discussed, because she can't ask her husband without revealing the plot. Of course, deep down, this represents another mild conflict over who's to wear the pants in the marriage, but some men like to be mothered a little. So long as the nagging isn't an obsession that poisons their whole relationship, I don't go to the lengths of having them both come to the office for a discussion.

After the wars between the sexes, there are the wars between generations. Dominating mothers and submissive husbands sometimes raise submissive sons. In my practice, a common example is provided by the mother who brings her son to the office, gives his history, asks about his diet, shots, and sleeping hours, and scoops up his prescriptions—and he's 20 years old! I used to make these mothers stay in the waiting room until I discovered that one couldn't treat the puppet without permission of the puppeteer. Then, too, I discovered that when I was effective in releasing Sonny from bondage (usually through mobilization of a detached father), Mother went into a depression. Since the treatment for *that* was to replace her son's affection with that of another male, I came right back to Father again. With this near-perfect example of the fact that one sick person in a family usually indicates the presence of others, I've now learned to get all three of them in (usually separately) and tell each in turn what I think the trouble is. Then if the parents kick the son out, and if Father stays home more with Mother, and if Mother gets a job working with other people's children, they all live happily ever after. Sometimes, after many years, they even get over their initial resentment of me.

The reverse of the mother-dominated son is the aged parent who is dominated by his children. When the old leader of the wolf pack gets weak, the young pups fight for his crown. Humans are more subtle, but the same sort of struggle sometimes takes place, and then I get the feeling that the battle rages all over the hospital room and me. A common example (and it's getting more frequent) is the case of a senile parent who is no longer able to live alone. None of the children wants "Mother *put* in a nursing home" (they phrase it as though nursing homes were jails), but no one particularly wants to take her into *his* home, either. Usually, she'll end up with the youngest daughter, and usually there'll be no discussion of compensation for that daughter. She and her husband will assume that they are to get the major chunk of the old girl's estate—though this thought never gets into the open.

Eventually, Mother breaks a hip, and nursing home care

becomes a necessity. Youngest daughter feels guilty about letting Mother fall, and empathically she suffers her mother's pain. On a deeper level, she is ashamed that she is glad to be relieved of Mother's care and fearful that her sacrifices will be forgotten if Mother lives a long time. Her siblings will fear that a prolonged illness may consume the estate and will feel guilt over not having shared the burdens of her care. The situation is ripe for an explosion of misdirected feelings, and an inept doctor can be an apt target.

My solution is to call a family conference—Sundays are best—with all the sibs *and their spouses* present. (In my experience the wife of the eldest son can be the most guilt-ridden and grasping of them all.) And then we talk frankly about money, wills, powers of attorney, and—if necessary—guilt feelings. It doesn't do much for my patient, but it keeps a family together in a time of crisis and saves me a whale of a lot of grief from angry telephone calls. Usually I manage to get a cash settlement for the youngest daughter that's large enough to make the sibs feel noble yet small enough to leave her some of the rewards of generosity and self-sacrifice.

Sometimes a family is so fragmented that the grown children don't speak to each other. Then, if Mother gets sick, each member can be expected to call independently for a report on her condition. Even in close families the calls are sometimes duplicated. I start by saying, "Your sister has already called, and as I told her . . ." If that doesn't get the message across, the next day I go on to: "I've already discussed this with your sister—would you mind calling her for the information?" In extreme cases, I've said, "Look, you're a large family. I expect to talk to at least one member of the family every day, but too many calls are coming in. How about your designating one member of the family to make the daily call, and then I'll have more time to spend with your mother?" Otherwise, I have an understandable tendency to give shorter and gruffer answers to each caller until the whole family is alienated.

One of the philosophies of medical care with which I violently disagree holds that, in cases where tough decisions must be made, the responsibility should be dumped on the relatives' shoulders. Recently, newspapers headlined the case of a father who had to decide whether to have his son's remaining eye removed to lessen his chances of retinoblastoma. Less dramatically, I hear of doctors saying, "Your mother probably should have her gallbladder out, but at her age there's some risk; we'll let you decide."

The relatives are thus forced to make decisions from imperfect knowledge of the facts, with a judgment colored by personal emotions. And if things go wrong, they may be left with almost intolerable guilt. Whenever I'm unable to make a tough decision, I dump it in the lap of a consultant, not a relative.

There's also the problem of the relative (almost always a wife or mother) who wants to come between the doctor and the patient. She may subconsciously want to be a patient or a doctor herself, or she may simply be so involved in the patient's ego that she thinks of him as an extension of herself. These are touchy situations, and I don't think pat formulas can be given. If the doctor bluntly insists on having the patient all to himself he may create antagonism in both patient and relative. On the other hand, he may make himself a hero. (Or a fool: Once I arbitrarily excluded a man's wife from the interview room only to discover that he was aphasic, whereupon I had to eat humble pie in order to get a history.) Certainly a normal male of almost any age will resent having a woman barge in and give his history, grab his prescriptions, and flounce out with a promise to see that he behaves. When he doesn't resent this sort of treatment it tells a lot about him.

I try to call patients from the waiting room myself. In the case of adolescents I pleasantly tell the mother that I'll want to visit with her later, which usually puts her back in her seat. If it's a husband I watch his face: If he looks distressed as she rises, I ask to see him alone. On the other hand, if he asks if it's all right for his wife to come along I accede freely. Once in the consultation room, if she starts giving the history for him, or disagrees with his history, or if they get to wrangling over nonessential points, I pretend the history is over, take him into the examining room, suggest that she'll be more comfortable in the waiting room, and then finish the history when he's undressed and on the table.

One should also beware of suspicions aroused in the person who is left out. A wife sitting in the waiting room can easily believe her husband is blaming her for his troubles; a patient in a hospital bed who hears his family talking with the doctor in the corridor will be quite sure that his condition is too grim for him to bear—probably cancerous.

As a general rule, the longer I practice the more comfortable and productive I find myself when I share my patient with his family. The family is the basic unit of our social life. Much as a doctor may wish to deal with his patients as isolated individuals —perhaps even to "father" or "mother" them himself—he'll have to recognize that family relationships are longer and stronger. If he can use them productively they can be potent forces for change. If he runs counter to the family, no matter how good his intentions, his science and his skill may be wasted.

CHAPTER 15

Pitfalls in Referrals and Consultations

One of the more admirable aspects of our profession is our tradition of deferring to a colleague's opinion when things appear to be going askew. I don't mean the internist-to-surgeon consult: There's nothing unusual about calling in an expert in another field. I mean the increasingly popular internist-to-internist or, in small towns, G.P.-to-G.P. referrals. Then, too, in partnerships and groups a great deal of less formal collaboration goes on.

This meeting of two minds with separate thoughts not only protects against malpractice suits and cross-fertilizes the doctors' intellects, it's almost always reassuring to the patient and his relatives, too.

That is, provided everyone understands what's going on. One large medical society reported that 40 per cent of all complaints reaching its grievance committee stemmed from patients who received bills for consultations they hadn't authorized. Doctors apparently tangle over consultations, too, because a recent MEDICAL ECONOMICS survey of doctors showed that one-third of the respondents had dropped at least one consultant from their lists in the last year.

To call in a competitor to review one's work requires a high order of generosity, maturity, and scientific objectivity, so it's not surprising that human emotions often get in the way of the elegant ethics spelled out by the A.M.A. Considering that the already-strained doctor-patient contract spreads to a doctor-patient-doctor contract, it's easy to understand how interpersonal nerves get jangled—especially if the relatives jump into the arena, too.

Let's look at the start of these situations, when only the first two parties are on the scene. Sometimes regulations require consultations—abortions and sterilization operations are a common example—and here no great problems arise because the consultant is expected to concur promptly with what the attending and his patient have in mind and then get out.

The problems come when the primary doctor has either lost the patient's faith or failed to get it in the first place. Generally, it's not hard to tell when this happens: The patient looks unhappy, the relatives have endless questions about particulars of the case, and the nurses start telegraphing warning signals.

The experienced, sensitive (and lucky) doctor will see this coming a long way off and ask for a consultation at least one day before the relatives suggest it. Usually people are painfully reluctant to bring up the matter of a consultant because they fear "hurting the doctor's feelings." By the creepy way they sidle up to the subject you can tell they're pretty embarrassed and frightened of a possible explosion.

At this point, there's only one way to get out—and that's graciously: "Why of course, I'd be delighted. I've been wanting to share the responsibility for some time, but I wasn't sure *you'd* be in favor of it." If one can keep from looking like a little boy caught with his hand in the jam jar, it may just come off.

My formula for avoiding all this embarrassment on both sides runs something like this:

"Mary, I wonder if you'd let me spend some of your money on a consultant? As far as I can tell, everything's going pretty well, but two heads are always better than one, and maybe another man could find a way to get you better faster. Anyway, I'd sleep better with the reassurance of another opinion."

Once consultation has been agreed upon, there comes the matter of selecting the man for the job, assuming a choice is available. Since the attending has the tacit responsibility of carrying out the consultant's recommendations, he'll want a man he trusts. But if he names him too eagerly, doubts will be sparked in the relatives' minds that the two are in cahoots, particularly if the consultant is bland and voluble in his reassurances. This is quite apt to happen; it wouldn't be human of the attending to be attracted to a consultant who often disagreed with his medical views.

On the other hand, if the relatives are left to name the consultant, they will occasionally pick a charlatan or a specialist of more age than wisdom, or one whose vast popularity is fed solely by a flamboyant bedside manner. In such cases the attending has the sticky chore of disparaging a colleague with every certainty that his words will be misquoted as they're spread.

To obviate these hazards, I give a choice of three men that I think will work well with the patient, after this fashion:

"If you don't have somebody in mind, I'd recommend Dr. A, Dr. B, or Dr. C. There are many other good men available too, but for problems like yours I'd suggest one of those three. Naturally, I'm going to continue to be your doctor as I have been in the past, although if you find you like your new doctor better, I'll have to give you up."

Said with a wink and a smile, this last usually leads to some mutual exchanges of endearments that are reassuring to us both.

When they're available, the suggestion of three possible consultants seems about right. Too many names occasion perplexity, while too few suggest collusion. If the patient says, "I don't know, Doctor; anyone you say is fine with me," I think out loud, listing some good features of each of the three, and then softly settle on the one I've wanted all along.

The entrance of the consultant ushers out the one-to-one doctor-patient relationship of the past, maybe for good. It's kind and generous to let the new man go as far as he and the patient like in taking the case over. Particularly when there are emotional problems, he's going to have to establish rapport in order to be helpful. In many cases he may establish a firmer bond than the patient has ever had with his frantic, hard-pressed G.P.

When I'm the consultant, I like freedom. In the old days, the referring man was supposed to meet the consultant at the bedside, introduce him to the patient, stand by during the exam, and then introduce him to the relatives for the final act in this stylized playlet. I've done some consultations under those circumstances and I must say I was most uncomfortable—trying to see the case for myself with the family physician hovering around, trying to uncover his mistakes diplomatically, and realizing all the while that I was taking up an hour or two of his time for which he could not charge. My personal preference is that he put everything he knows about the case on the chart (where it should be, unless it's highly confidential or slanderous) and let me pick my own time to see the patient in solitude. And I don't like to try to write a cogent report while the attending is chattering in my ear about golf.

Naturally, as the consulting, I expect that the attending has told the patient I'll be coming (without telling him exactly when) and that I'll expect to be paid (without telling him exactly how much). While I try to see every hospital consultation within 24 hours, I like to select the hour.

One of my peeves is the casual type who catches me in the hospital and says something like, "Good, I was looking for an internist (meaning '*any* internist'). Come up and look at my patient, will you? *I* don't think we need a consultant, but the relatives are on my back, and I'd like you to tell them everything's going all right." Nor is there a warm spot in my heart for the man who temporizes all week and decides on an emergency consultation on Sunday or my day off.

I have little use for the possessive doctor who fouls up a case, calls in help, and then expects the helper to hoodwink the patient into believing things were fine in the first place. Not only is the consultant asked to delude the patient but, if the consultant does a good job, the patient is left wondering why he should pay a second doctor who contributed nothing.

It seems to me that the first doctor is obligated to praise his colleague to the skies and tell the patient how much the consultation benefited both of them. I can't recall ever knowing of a referring doctor who did so, but I'll bet it would do a lot to improve his stature in the relatives' eyes. Only big men can be humble. Unfortunately, it's the defensive, insecure doctor who most often gets himself into the hot water of needing consultation or having it urged on him, since patients and their relatives tend to accept a doctor at his own valuation.

Some men build up a large consulting practice by seldom disagreeing with the attending man, while praising him heartily to the patient. Others take the "cold fish" approach, emphasizing science but not art and communicating with the patient as little as possible. In any event, if one has to depend on consultations for a living he must know his referrings well, and artfully vary his approach as indicated. While the patient's needs should come first, a doctor in internal medicine or pediatrics who is too artful at pleasing referred patients can shortly find himself out of the consultation business.

One of the failings of my consultants that disturbs my relations with my patients is the sending of late or incomplete reports. This is particularly a trait of the big medical centers and clinics which have never, so far as I know, mastered the challenge of getting a letter dictated, typed, read, corrected, and in the mail in 24 hours. It puts me in an uncomfortable position when a patient calls to get the results of his consultation and no report has come. If anything happens to the patient in that interim I'll be handicapped by not wanting to change treatment until the report arrives.

I'm probably wrong, but failure to get patients to come back to me is not one of the consultation problems that bug me. I won't say I was happy the time a doctor at the Big Clinic referred my patient to my competitor in town—a man who had trained at Big Clinic where I had not. But if Big Clinic decides to take over treatment of a problem I've sent them, I think that's up to them and the patient. Somehow, thinking of people as permanently "my patients" seems to me a degree of possessiveness that borders on an invasion of their rights. Furthermore, I doubt seriously that a man can be an effective therapist if he feels too strongly about holding onto patients; it makes him too vulnerable to their manipulations.

Psychiatrists have written numerous articles on the proper selection and preparation of patients for psychotherapy, as though that were a unique problem in medicine. Now that Hollywood has made psychiatric treatment a status symbol, I have little trouble getting patients to go for such help. But I *do* have a great deal of trouble getting any report back. Some psychiatrists feel that any communication they get is privileged, even from the attending doctor, but if I'm the man who gets called to the home to give a shot for the sick headache, I want to know its psychodynamics, to say nothing of what tranquilizers the patient is getting. Apparently psychiatrists do have a problem with doctors who hoodwink patients into thinking they're going to see a neurologist instead of a psychiatrist. I've had occasional alcoholics sent to me for what the patient and I both assumed was a medical consultation, only to be asked later by the attending why I didn't talk to the man about his drinking problem. Certainly honest, frank communication with both consultant and patient is the best policy.

But in general, I don't think the psychiatrists have any larger problems as consultants than the rest of us: broken appointments, prejudiced patients, insufficient information from the attending, inordinate expectations of miraculous cures, diagnoses hopelessly snarled by therapy, and bad collection of bills make the referral part of my practice my least satisfying work.

CHAPTER 16

Getting Along With Third Parties

In medicine the term "third party" usually refers to a silent partner—or "intruder"—in the doctor-patient relationship who pays some, or all, of the bill. In a sense, the patient still pays through taxes or insurance premiums, but he often overlooks this fact in his headlong rush to get all of the services he can. Doctors overlook the fact, too, when they order extra tests and treatments because the patient is "covered by insurance." Rising costs are reflected in rising taxes and premiums.

Peculiarly, both doctor and patient often react to the aid of these remote and impersonal agencies with rancor, as though the intimacy of their relations were spoiled by the intrusion of such indirect payment. Doctors resent the filling out of forms, even though in an efficient office all that is required of them is a signature. If the insurer questions the service, an explosion occurs. Popular articles are written on how a doctor successfully "puts down" an insurance company or government agency.

Patients show their hostility by trying to bilk the carrier (with or without collusion of the attending physician) and by siding with the doctor in cursing the paper work, delay, and complexity of obtaining a settlement.

Granted that clerks and bureaucrats can pull some astounding boners at times, it's always seemed to me immature to kick the goose that lays the guaranteed egg. While it's possible that I may not approve of the agency my patient has enlisted to pay my bill, my interest in his welfare demands that I cooperate with it. Besides, I should be grateful that payment of at least part of my bill *is* guaranteed.

Doctors who cannot view third parties in this fashion—who get a 20-point rise in systolic pressure whenever a governmental or insurance form appears—would do well to delegate all these matters to an aide or else to join a clinic. We don't improve our public image when we go into a frenzy over petty threats to our sovereignty.

Nor do we impress our clientele by waiting months to fill out those forms. Patients worry about unpaid bills, even when the insurance company is responsible for them. Carriers are wonderfully efficient in meeting their obligations to us, and it seems to me we're equally obligated to be prompt and cooperative.

Now I'd like to stretch the term "third parties" to include a discussion of other situations in which commercial and governmental agencies enter the doctor-patient relationship.

For example, life insurance companies purchase case summaries on my patients and hire me to examine applicants. One difficult situation arises when I'm asked to do a life insurance examination on one of my own patients. Let's say I know the man needs the insurance badly because he has a lot of children but no estate, while his wife has previously complained to me that he's an alcoholic. When I get to the question on the blank about alcohol consumption, the man says he's never drunk to excess.

Or, as I've had happen, suppose a patient who is due for his regular physical exam asks me to do an insurance exam at the same time, letting the carrier pay part of the bill. For purposes of his regular exam he should give me every little symptom he can dredge up, but for the insurance company he'll want to report that everything's just great.

In both these situations I've found the best solution is prevention—I refuse to do insurance exams on my own patients, carefully explaining to them the conflict of interest involved.

Dr. Michael J. Halberstam has raised several knotty questions about the conflicts that arise when third parties ask for information about patients.* For example, there are the matters of epileptics under good control who need driver's licenses, or an employment questionnaire on a patient who had a problem with sexual perversion some years ago. One can draw ever finer lines until the most honest physician would be tempted to tell white lies. Yet, if something happened and the truth came out in court, the doctor would have only the feeblest defense. And there's growing danger that continued disclosure of information to third parties, not only in such cases but in the growing number in which disclosure is legally mandatory (battered children, rape, attempted suicide, venereal disease in many states), will eventually make our patients afraid to confide in us. Some day we may regret not having preserved for our offices the status of the confessional.

On the brighter side there are those stimulating contacts with insurance carriers that, to me, are among the most challenging parts of my practice. I refer to those situations in which a patient is sent to a doctor other than his own for disability evaluation, life insurance examination, pre-employment health appraisal, or a determination of his eligibility for pension or compensation.

---

*MEDICAL ECONOMICS, May 15, 1967.

This is an increasingly important field of medicine. Some doctors specialize in it, and almost all G.P.s, internists, and orthopods dabble in it.

Here, the usual doctor-patient relationship turns almost 180 degrees. In ordinary doctor-patient relations it is presumed (not always correctly) that the patient is motivated to be cooperative and accurate. In these special relationships, on the other hand, the converse must be assumed: that the patient sees me as standing between him and an insurance policy, a job, or a big fat compensation award. Initially, I'm suspected of being a hireling of "the company," and antagonism is taken for granted.

I enjoy these examinations because they require far more skill than any others—skill in disarming the patient's suspicion, in evaluating his history, in doing a physical examination that will disclose things he may be hiding (like the "completely" disabled man with a double row of calluses on both hands), and in rendering a report intelligible to a layman. Further, collections for this kind of medical service are 100 per cent; one can even charge for broken appointments.

True, it's all diagnosis and no therapy, unless helping to end a protracted case and thus to halt the attendant compensation neurosis counts.

To begin, one must guard against trying to make findings that will please the purchaser. An ethical, honest doctor should have nothing to do with an agency that attempts to influence his decisions, and he mustn't feel that his livelihood will be threatened if he makes too many unfavorable reports.

And that's exactly where I start my relationship with the patient. I point out to him with all the sincerity I can muster that I have no personal interest in the outcome of my exam; in most cases I don't make the decision as to whether he gets what he's after, and usually I don't even hear what the decision is. "In any event," I say with a smile, "I get my pay.

"Our job—yours and mine," I continue, "is to get down on paper as thorough and accurate a report of the true state of affairs as we can, so that someone can make a fair decision. The company that hires me wants to do what's right—if they didn't, I wouldn't work for them. If you're entitled to this award, we want you to get it. The reason you're here is that it's their duty to get a true, objective picture of what's going on. Chances are that if you and I do our job well the decision will be made in a hurry and you'll find out where you stand. If we don't, it may drag on for months or even end in court."

This makes a lot of sense to most people, and the atmosphere usually thaws considerably, especially since I do my best to pour on the charm. Of course, I never let him know how I personally feel about his petition, because the outcome might be contrary to my feelings, and the discrepancy could get a lot of people, including me, into trouble.

When the history is over, I really spike his guns by asking, "Now, is there anything else you can think of that we should put down here that might help your case?" Then he can never say that I wasn't thorough or didn't give him a chance to tell the whole story. And I take the history in my own handwriting as he gives it, trying to use his own words as much as possible. Seeing me write as he talks will convince him that I'm not leaving anything out, and direct quotations are very helpful when it comes to court testimony.

Actually, I write the first part of my report as I take the history, then dictate the physical exam, lab reports, and conclusion while he's dressing, so that most of the report is ready for typing by the time he's left the office. By the next morning it's usually on the desk of the purchaser. The companies, like any referring agency, always appreciate prompt, accurate service, pleased patients, and immediate, understandable reports.

With this system, it's a rare patient who doesn't thank me as he leaves—some even ask if they can transfer to my care. (That, of course, is absolutely impossible under any circumstances because of the charges of conflict of interest and patient-stealing that would result.)

There are a few things to look out for, I've found. For one thing, there's really a fourth party in these relationships, and that's the patient's own physician, who will probably hear if any disparagement of his care is expressed. Rarely, he may not know why you're seeing his patient, and leap to some unpleasant conclusions.

It's important to know that your report will probably be available to the patient and others since—except for life insurance examinations—there are no privileged communication safeguards in these relationships. In the case of compensation exams, one copy of the report will always be forwarded to the patient's lawyer and may well be read in open court. Many doctors have a compulsion to vent their hostility through gratuitously insulting descriptions of a patient in the physical exam report. Even when done in privileged circumstances, this practice can be dangerous. I once received photostatic records of a patient described in his Florida doctor's records as "a real Caspar Milquetoast." The description may have been accurate, but the patient was my uncle and he'd been given the photostatic records in an unsealed envelope.

In reporting to third parties it's best to avoid opinions and stick to facts. It isn't necessary to say that you believe a patient has a compensation neurosis or is faking or malingering—simply present the evidence and let others draw the obvious conclusions. For example, one can say: "Despite his history of living a bed-to-bathroom existence for the last year, he has corns and thick calluses on both feet" or, "While he limped badly in the office, he was observed to walk briskly and normally to his car."

Ordinarily, since no treatment is involved, one might think

that third-party exams are immune to malpractice risks; unfortunately this isn't so. As noted by Howard Hassard in the book "Medical Malpractice: Risks, Protection, Prevention,"° courts have recently given decisions that make a doctor liable for mistakes committed during pre-employment exams even though the usual doctor-patient relationship is absent. Mr. Hassard also points out that a doctor is now legally responsible for seeing that the patient is informed when he uncovers a serious condition in the course of a third-party exam. The moral responsibility has been there for some time, while the ethics have yet to be spelled out.

For example, I've several times had the experience of finding diabetes in a man who is alleging that his work brought on a heart attack. Even though my employer, the workmen's compensation insurance carrier, might like to discredit the testimony of the patient's physician by springing this new knowledge while he's on the witness stand, the patient's welfare is the paramount consideration.

Still, it would be wrong to notify the patient in a way that would reflect on his doctor. And, since I'm working for the insurance company, I have no right to divulge information without its permission. But the solution is easy. If the patient is intelligent and there is no reason to avoid an informal approach, I tell him that we seem to have picked up a suggestion that he might have diabetes and that he should call his doctor to have it checked as soon as possible. Otherwise, the formal procedure is to call the company's representative and ask him to relay the information to the patient's doctor, or offer to do it yourself with the representative's permission.

The situation is tougher when the examination discloses that the attending physician has made a wrong diagnosis, is grossly

---

°Medical Economics Book Division, Inc., 1966.

incompetent, or has committed malpractice. Here there are so many conflicting responsibilities and relationships that I just throw in the sponge, do nothing, and feel guilty about it. I wish I could say that the situation is rare, but it isn't. In my experience, many times when a man sues for compensation because of prolonged disability he might better be suing his doctor for malpractice.

All in all, my experience with third parties—including governmental welfare and Social Security representatives—has been most favorable. Once I've communicated my problem to the right person, I've almost invariably found that his concern for the welfare of the patient is not exceeded by mine, while his suggested solution to my dilemma is usually far superior to mine because he's met the same situation many times before.

CHAPTER 17

When Your Patient Is a Doctor

Since Hippocrates, medical tradition has required doctors to take care of other doctors and their families free of charge. That may have seemed a wonderful idea in Hippocrates's time, but more recently this medical free-loading has resulted in some of the most difficult, painful, and unsatisfactory relationships in all medicine. From what I've heard at cocktail parties, there's little doubt that our wives would agree.

In June, 1967, the A.M.A. Judicial Council attempted to correct the situation with the odd pronouncement that, if the recipient "insists upon payment, the physician need not be embarrassed to accept a fee for his services." Far from alleviating the pain of these encounters, I predict this new edict will only make things more difficult. Certainly the physician will undergo some embarrassment as he tries to discover whether his patient is really insisting or simply making a gesture.

An additional moral complication comes with the new "usual-and-customary" fee provisions for governmental and Blue Shield benefits. Many doctors subscribed to Blue Shield in the past so that their colleagues could at least draw pay for any hospital care rendered them. Under the new provision, however, a doctor will be theoretically dishonest to accept such payments because the usual-and-customary fee for the care of doctors and their families is zero.

Under any system, it's difficult to care for (or be cared for by) close friends. We routinely refuse to take care of relatives for this reason, but almost never refuse to care for a colleague who may be emotionally closer to us than some of our relatives.

Let's look, first, at some of the distortions of the normal doctor-patient relationship that I feel when I have another physician as a patient:

• I'm flattered that such a medically sophisticated person has chosen to depend on me.

• I'm afraid that I may not be equal to that trust; that he'll be quick to perceive my deficiencies, particularly in his own field of medicine; and that I'll be unable to use my usual techniques on him because he'll react differently and see through my deceptions or manipulations.

• I'm embarrassed for him because I find it easy to see him as an extension of myself, and I know that a doctor is not supposed to join "them"—the ranks of the diseased and infirm. We both know that doctors are not supposed to get sick; doctors are not supposed to be neurotic; doctors are not supposed to have normal emotions.

• I don't believe he will be honest with me, because I would find it very hard to be completely honest with a colleague; I don't believe he's going to follow my orders well because *I* wouldn't if the situation were reversed.

• I don't really believe in the efficacy of all the measures I advise, but I like my patients to believe in them so they'll feel they've been helped. The chances are that my doctor-patient won't believe in my remedies any more than I do, and there goes a lot of my magic power to be helpful.

• Now that this man has become my patient, I can never let down and be an "ordinary" person when he's around. It's bad enough to have to play the role of a doctor when I'm out in public—now I'll have to do so when I'm at some of the medical social functions where I can ordinarily be more like my true self.

• I must be at least twice as good a doctor to this man as to my rank-and-file patients because he's a more valuable person, being one of my set; because all the other members of my set will note and be critical if I let anything happen to him; because I want to convince him that being a nonpaying patient doesn't make him a second-class citizen here; because he'll notice it if I cut corners.

• I'm more comfortable treating laymen because I'm superior to them. It's much harder to deal with equals. Of course, the fact that he's petitioned me for help automatically gives me a certain degree of superiority to him.

And here are some of the things I feel when I'm a patient:

• I wish I could resign temporarily from the doctor ranks and be treated like everybody else, except better.

• I'm ashamed that I got sick; that I'm impotent over disease in myself when I'm supposed to be able to banish it from others; that I'm not able to treat myself. "Physician, heal thyself" now conflicts with the motto that "a doctor who cares for himself has a fool for a patient."

• I don't really trust any other doctor because I know that medical science is mostly guesswork and I know how many mistakes I've made. As a sick person I badly need to feel that this doctor is godlike, but I can't; I know him too well.

- I'd like to ask him if I have cancer, but I can't because it would be weak and neurotic for a doctor to fear death.
- I'm ashamed to have him discover my varicose veins or my pruritis ani or that hernia I've never had the courage to get fixed. If he *does* notice them, I hope he won't mention it.
- I'd like some medicine for pain, but I don't dare ask for it or he'll think I'm a sissy or an addict, or that I'm trying to run my own case. Doctors are supposed to make terrible patients, so I'll have to be especially docile.
- We'll be expected to give him a gift next Christmas, which will be embarrassing, because it won't be a gift but a token payment.
- Suppose he doesn't find out what's wrong? Suppose he comes up with a diagnosis or advice that I can't accept? How can I break off and go somewhere else or get a consultant?

And here's what I think doctors' wives feel:

- When I married a doctor I thought I'd have the best medical attention in the world; that my husband would give me even more sympathy and concern than he does his patients, and would get the best specialists for me. Yet when I'm sick he acts as though he were upset; as though I were taking advantage of him for free advice; as though he didn't want to hear about it.
- I used to think that doctors were smart and never made mistakes, but I've heard so many cocktail stories of what goes on in hospitals I'd be scared to death to go to one, and my husband talks so much about other doctors' deficiencies that I can't think of any I could trust.
- When the children are sick, I'd like to have my husband treat them—he's a doctor, after all. But he just glances at them and says it's nothing. If I call the pediatrician I'll look terribly foolish if it's really nothing, and besides it would be disloyal to go behind my husband's back.

• I don't feel right about being a nonpaying patient. We can afford to pay our way, and if I were paying for service I'd feel free to ask for it. Sometimes I feel as though the kids and I don't get anything like the medical attention that other people do. I could be half dead and nobody would know it. I'd like to be able to have regular exams and take the children in for camp and school exams without feeling guilty about imposing.

• I wish I could pay off our obligations with a check. I never know what to give for gifts—doctors have everything they need.

• If I needed an operation I'd like to go to the best surgeon in the country, but I couldn't because all our friends who are surgeons would be hurt.

All in all, there's a lot of insecurity when doctors and their families get sick. Some of it is inevitable. I suppose lawyers are scared to death when they get personally involved with the law, and maybe plumbers panic when the pipes in their own houses break.

But I think we could do better than we often do as doctors, doctor-patients, and doctor's family-patients. Here are some improvements I'd like to suggest:

When an internist, pediatrician, or gynecologist accepts responsibility for a doctor or members of a doctor's family, he should feel obligated to call them in for yearly routine checkups, recognizing their reluctance to come otherwise. On the first visit I tell each such person who comes to me: "I'm flattered to be asked to care for you—it's a great privilege. I make only these stipulations: You must see me yearly when I call you in; you must call me as you would a doctor under other circumstances—early in the course of the disease; and you must feel free to leave me for another doctor any time you wish."

When a doctor's wife is a patient I add the further suggestion that she call me directly whenever she's concerned about her

health. Lest this sound like encouraging disloyalty to her husband, I say something like: "As you've probably already discovered, we doctors have a peculiar emotional reaction to illness in
members of our own family. If you are worried about yourself,
I'd suggest that you tell me about it instead of telling Jim. Naturally, if it's important, we'll tell him immediately."

In exchange for the lost "magic" and faith of the usual doctor-
patient relationship I take advantage of a doctor-patient's medical knowledge and make him a part-time consultant in his own
case. It's foolish to treat him "like anyone else," because he isn't. I
let my doctor-patients see their own X-rays or X-ray reports and
all laboratory reports and direct them to the best medical litera-
ture on their disorders. This doesn't mean they run their own
cases, but when they know as much about the diseases as I do
there shouldn't be much difficulty in reaching a consensus.

Anyway, when any doctor is sick enough to be hospitalized,
I request consultation—with another internist if it's a medical
problem, with two surgeons if it's surgical, and so on, so that
there'll be at least two minds (plus the patient's!) pondering
every problem.

Better yet, I try to transfer him to the "Big Medical Center,"
because they'll have more magic down there, their nurses won't
be afraid of him as ours are, and he'll be able to give a more
honest history than he would to me. They might even be able to
do more for him.

When doctors are patients it would be nice if they'd forget the
role of doctor and be "just folks." Many of them do very well at
this—actually, the professional patient who bothers me is less the
one who throws his weight around than the one who hesitates to
ask for even ordinary amounts of care for fear he'll be taking
advantage of his position.

The matter of feeling guilty about being free-loaders is very
easily solved by giving presents, but not at Christmas—it's fool-

ish to pretend that a token payment is a true gift. And it's risky to give a popular doctor a present without checking with his wife or secretary as to his wants. The best gift of all, I think, is a gift certificate at a department store in his wife's name (so he won't have to take time to shop). The amount should be large enough to enable the donor's family to call for service in the future without feeling guilty. I'd suggest at least 50 per cent of your estimate of his usual bill. If you think he's the honest sort who will report any gift over $25 as taxable income (as he's supposed to), better increase it to 60 or 75 per cent—at least give until the guilt feelings go.

In my opinion the A.M.A. Judicial Council would have done a great deal to solve the fee problem by saying that doctors and their dependents are entitled to a 25 to 50 per cent reduction in medical fees, whether from psychoanalysts, Medicare, or Blue Shield. That way, everybody would be almost satisfied about money and we'd be left with only the other emotional pains of these relationships.

CHAPTER 18

The Cheerful Practice Is a Limited One

Is it ethical to turn sick people away? There's a school of sanctimony which holds that all doctors are divinely called to minister to mankind until they die of exhaustion. That puts a lot of guilt on those who do less.

I don't have any objection to a man living and breathing medical practice if his family can stand it; I do object to his claiming greater dedication to Hippocrates or a lesser degree of laziness than I possess—even if it's true. By public handwringing over our large workloads, we've discouraged a lot of fine boys from going into medicine. Few laymen know that almost half of all doctors are on salaried 40-to-50 hour workweeks. And I see no reason why any man can't do general practice for a mere 40 hours a week and still feel he's a good doctor—even a superior doctor. Dedication is for martyrs, and martyrs are very fine people but I wouldn't want my daughter to marry one.

A rested, relaxed, unharassed doctor is the only one who can practice the brand of medicine we've been discussing. The man who tries to please all pleases few; by failing to cull his flock, limit his practice load, and preserve his recreation time he loses the joy in production that characterizes the happy doctor.

I used to have the naive belief that the better a doctor was, the larger his practice would be. In a market of limited demand for care and an unlimited supply of doctors that would be true—if people were machines. Since doctors and patients are human and in most areas today we have almost unlimited demand but a limited supply of doctors, the better doctors are often those who keep their practices small enough to keep themselves and their patients healthy and happy.

Theoretically, if the demands for care are unrestricted, any doctor could work to the limits of exhaustion and still not run out of patients. Yet every practice levels off at some point. My thesis is that a doctor either limits his practice or his practice limits itself, willy-nilly. The problem for medicine as a whole is that the doctor who refuses to prune his practice lets it grow wildly until it outgrows its blood supply—his time and concern. When patients go elsewhere because their former doctor has become too busy, it's bad for our public relations and inefficient for over-all care. Such doctors remind me of a man who buys a country estate because he likes to grow things, and then becomes so busy earning money to pay for it that he doesn't have time to tend his flowers and trees.

A large practice doesn't convince me that the proprietor is popular or good. It's more apt to suggest that he's so insecure that he can't summon the courage to say No, or that he is undisciplined and disordered. I've even identified a few who appear to be simply greedy—who seem to want all the patients and all the money they can get.

Let's look at some of the factors that limit a man's practice when he doesn't:

If he doesn't work by appointments, the long waits in the

waiting room will drive out the busy, the impatient, and the suffering, leaving for his practice the idle, passive, and healthy.

If he does work by appointments, his appointments will progressively be scheduled farther ahead, then closer together. We've already discussed the disadvantages of scheduling too far ahead (Chapter 9). While increased efficiency could enable most of us to see more people in less time, there comes a point of diminishing returns at which everybody—the doctor, his aides, and the patient—gets unhappy.

Suppose he raises prices? The character of his clientele may change, but chances are the volume will grow just the same.

Specialization is an excellent practice limiter, especially if one goes into one of the overpopulated fields such as general surgery. G.P.s who are overloaded can cut out obstetrics or pediatrics. But it's hard for a man established in practice to develop a new specialty. In the old days he simply changed the sign out front to announce that he was now an allergist or a proctologist or what not. Now, increasingly, he needs specialty training to get hospital recognition of his new status.

How about adding a partner? That's probably the worst solution of all for reducing a man's workload. If the partner is any good at all, he'll soon attract more patients. It's true that the senior partner will have more assurance of freedom from interruption during his time off. But he'll have less time off altogether because he'll work more than twice as hard handling unfamiliar patients during his periods of covering for the other man. Besides, he'll be less apt to take time off for fear of not carrying his half of the load.

Even his vacations will get him in deeper. When a solo practitioner takes a vacation, he returns to his regular workload—or if he stays away long enough his load may even be slightly reduced because some patients have tried other doctors and liked them better. But as noted, when a partner takes a vacation the other man works more than twice as hard. Just as this second man is about to drop from exhaustion they switch places. Now the senior partner expends all the benefits of *his* vacation filling in for the junior, while the junior needs his full vacation to recuperate from the larger-than-double load imposed during the senior's absence. So by the end of the summer they're back to normal— except that they've picked up a few more patients because they've kept their doors open continuously while the solo man was shut down.

Surveys show clearly that doctors in partnerships work longer hours than doctors in solo practice. The virtues of partnership practice are that patients find service more readily available and the partners make a higher hourly wage. Reduction of workload doesn't happen under ordinary circumstances.

Some men limit their practices by spending longer periods in being unavailable. If in town, they become hard to find because of an unlisted home telephone, or more days off, or being out on the golf course. Better yet, they take longer vacations or spend more time attending medical meetings. Getting to be a wheel in a state or national society works pretty well, too. I once met a man who claimed he had to see 80 patients a day because he was the only doctor for his whole county. Later, he said that his A.M.A. obligations kept him away from his office one-fifth of the time. I had to wonder at his naive belief that people in his county had no alternative sources of medical care.

Although it can't be measured, I suspect the foremost limiter of practice is almost entirely subconscious, because I find myself doing it. That's simply to be less satisfying when patients are burdensome and more satisfying when they're scarce. It's not hard to discover what a patient is after: If I withhold or deny it, he'll leave in time. Mostly, he'll be after a warm welcome and sympathy, so all I have to do is freeze him out with a cold professional manner. On those days when the phone rings constantly, when emergencies and consultation requests are popping up in several different hospitals, and when every minute of the schedule is crowded with two minutes of work, it's not hard to be abrupt with silly neurotics suffering "imaginary" ills. But the ills of those people are perfectly real to them. They're legitimate patients, and they shouldn't have to suffer the consequences of my busyness.

The only way I can possibly take care of people well, willingly, and promptly is to limit the numbers for whom I take responsibility. Any other solution creates even more unhappiness than the direct approach of cutting off new patients. Otherwise almost every practice must eventually reach a size at which it is no longer pleasurable for the doctor and serviceable to his clientele.

Everyone has limits. No one needs to feel guilty about avoiding overwork. I'll grant that a man who has been educated to be a doctor at a tax-supported school has obligations to those taxpayers, but that's not admitting that he's obliged to give up being human.

So the inevitable question comes: "What if everybody felt as you do? There wouldn't be enough doctors to go around." My answer to that is, "Don't blame *me* for the doctor shortage—being a doctor absolves me of that. Blame the people who didn't go into medicine, the planners who didn't plan, and the legislators who didn't legislate. Besides, 70 per cent of medical practice is nonessential to health and life, so we're a long way from a situation where people will die for want of care."

We've mentioned Horace Cotton's doctrine of "the cheerful fee"; now I'd like to delineate "the cheerful practice" as one in which the doctor can cheerfully give as much time as his patients are willing to purchase. When the doctor finds himself resenting patient demands, it's past time he called a halt.

In my own practice I recognized this point when my appointment book was regularly booked solid for a week ahead. Taking on more new people beyond that point would have been unfair to my family and to my established patients.

Initially it took courage to turn potential patients away: There were the fears of making people mad, of dumping heavier burdens on my colleagues, and of turning away business I might need some day. There were ego threats in no longer striving to have the largest practice in town and in transfusing my competitors with my overflow. And there's been stultification in dealing with the same people and problems over and over.

But I've found that the rewards of a pruned practice far outweigh the penalties.

So now if you call my office for an appointment the voice at the other end will ask whether we've seen you before as a patient. If you volunteer that one of your close relatives is a patient, we'll take you in, as we will if you've been referred by another doctor. Otherwise, the words are, "I'm sorry but we're not taking on new patients. If you don't have another doctor in mind, you might try Dr. ____." By suggesting the name of a new doctor in town, we avoid creating a panicky feeling that maybe no one is taking new patients anymore; we minimize the risk that the patient will call 15 or 20 offices and get the same response; and we get new doctors in town off to a fast (and grateful) start.

For a few years there were occasional times when we'd get caught up and would lower the floodgates a little to fill the appointment schedule. Of late years the reverse has been true: Despite the restrictions, my practice has grown slightly, so that at times it's necessary to turn down relatives and newcomers to town referred by out-of-town doctors. If that didn't hold the line, I'd consider dismissal of those oldtimers who make medical practice least pleasurable in our office. Five per cent of the patients cause 60 per cent of the headaches. As has been discussed (Chapter 11), these problem patients should be helped to reform before they're dumped upon someone else, but sometimes there's no substitute for the last-resort discipline of booting them out. I'd be sorry if there were very many cases of that sort in my practice, but I have, on rare occasions, asked patients to go elsewhere—much to their surprise and my eventual satisfaction. I'm sure it made them better patients for their next doctors, and it's done wonders for me.

My last rejectee was an obsessive cardiac neurotic who had had psychiatric treatment and knew his chest pains were fictitious, but who regularly called me at home several mornings a week to hear me say that it was all right for him to go to work that day. I tried everything: patience, confrontation, interpretation, reaching out, reaching in, and leaning backwards, but the annoyance was unabated. So one fine day I simply said, "I'm sorry, I no longer care to be your physician." Then I closed his file and went home a free man.

A doctor is neither legally, ethically, nor morally obligated to care for a patient if other help is available, but there are certain requirements for detaching. The law requires that suitable time be provided to find a new physician and that the patient not be abandoned during that interval. Since a rejected patient is likely to feel a strong desire to retaliate, it's wise to avoid suits for abandonment by sending written notice of the rejection by registered mail, return receipt requested.

Medical ethics require an offer of help in finding a new physician, who must be given a thorough summary of the patient's records. Common decency requires that the relationship be broken with dignity, tact, and kindness. In my book a doctor is really chicken if, as devices for driving off unwanted patients, he gives the dirty work to his nurse, hikes his fees beyond all reason, refuses to give necessary service, or schedules appointments months ahead.

I'm a firm believer in the doctrine that there can be no meaningful bond between two people in the absence of discipline.

Applied to medical practice, this means that a doctor must discipline his patients to be the kind of people he can enjoy serving. Smiling confrontation, motivating to change, application of peer pressure, breaking up games—all these are methods of leading patients into disciplined, healthy behavior.

But discipline of others requires discipline of self. In medical practice this means that the doctor must not permit himself to become overused, overextended, or overwrought.

CHAPTER 19

A Time for Truth

With dentists we share the burden of always trying to put ourselves out of business; with no one do we share the inevitability of losing, every time.

Oh, the surgeon, the pediatrician, the dermatologist, and the psychiatrist usually win because they play with stacked decks. But sooner or later, the general doctor loses every patient to death.

The measure of his science may be how long he's able to stave off the inevitable, but the measure of his art will be whether the rest of the family continues to come around for care after the funeral. A real pro may even pick up new patients by the way in which he handles these most difficult of all cases.

The reason is the modern myth that almost any disease can be cured if it's caught fast; that almost any ravage can be routed by rapid resort to the right remedy. When the relatives are sold on that myth, the bell is apt to toll for the poor old doctor. He may have seen his patient through tens of real crises and hundreds of imaginary ones; he may have been right every time he's seen his patient over many years. But he gets the blame, just the same, for not recognizing the last illness at its first faint stirring.

If he's lucky, that first symptom leads to a consultation outside his field. For example, a cough may lead my patient to a chest X-ray, which leads to a thoracic surgeon and a thoracotomy for lung cancer, followed by a radiologist and an oncologist. By the time I get him back (which will be pretty close to the *end* of time for him) he'll be glad to return to somebody who just listens to his problems without inflicting more pain on him. And the chances are good that his relatives will find one of those others upon whom they can hang the albatross of their guilt projections.

But when it's diabetes or a coronary or a stroke, there may be no hiding place for the L.M.D. Then the tricky task is to keep the faith.

Our relationships with the dying patient are distorted three ways: by our own reactions to failure and death, by the waning of the patient and the corresponding waxing of the relatives, and by the relatives' reactions to death in general and the demise of this individual in particular.

It has been said that one of the strong subconscious motivations that lead men to a medical career is an inordinate fear of death. According to this theory, many of us stayed up nights mnemonically learning the cranial nerves in hopes of dimming the shadow of our own grim reaper under the lamp of knowledge. (If so, the hope was false: Doctors die a little younger than laymen of comparable background.)

Having searched the subterranean saccules of my psyche for many years, and having attended a few physicians to the near bank of the River Styx, I fail to find any unusually prominent fears of death in them or me. But maybe this nonchalance was acquired later.

I *have* identified in myself, and have seen in other doctors, a desire to withdraw from the dying patient—a reluctance to stick around and watch the grandfather clock take its last tock, coupled with a creeping decline in intimacy once death appears inevitable. But I think this is similar to the reaction a mechanic gets when he sees an engine worn beyond repair, or a dentist when he has to pull a tooth: It's a reaction to personal feelings of helplessness more than a personal horror of death.

Yet as many psychiatrists have pointed out, such withdrawal may come when the patient most needs intimacy and support.

When death nears, one of the foremost barriers to a warm relationship between doctor and patient is nurtured, I find, by those unfortunate collusions between doctors and relatives to hoodwink the patient into believing that all's well when it's not.

"Do you or don't you tell the dying patient?" is a tired subject for medical student and psychiatric bull-sessions. I'll not belabor it here except to report my belief that a doctor avoids discussing the possibility of death with his patients in proportion to the *doctor's* own discomfort with the subject, just as a Victorian parent avoids discussing sex with his children. Furthermore, deceit makes a pretty lousy foundation on which to erect a close relationship.

The possibility of death is in the mind of every hospitalized patient. If the doctor avoids the subject—if he holds sotto voce corridor colloquies with echelons of grave kinsmen—that fear approaches the panic of certainty.Worse yet is the doctor who lies unconvincingly, or one who becomes unnaturally solicitous.

(I once asked a banquet companion how she had felt during her numerous postoperative periods when her surgeon visited her bedside briefly and brusquely, if at all. "Fine," said she. "If he ever sat down and patted my hand I'd be scared to death; as long as he neglects me I know I'm recuperating on schedule.")

Given time, the human mind can adjust to great travail, so I've learned to give my dying patients the word as early as possible. Of course I don't put it *that* bluntly, but, rather, say something like this: "Fred, I'm very much afraid that you have Hodgkin's disease. That's a very serious, often fatal, disease of the lymph nodes. Fortunately, it's slow and there are several treatments that control it, sometimes for many years. If I were in your shoes, I'd want the best, so, if you agree, I'll send you to the University Hospital for consultation. Then I'll work with them to get your disease under control and keep it there as long as possible."

It's extraordinary how much closer I am to dying patients and they to me since I've learned the virtues of being honest. In the old days I used to keep visits to a minimum for fear they'd pop the "fatal?" question; and I could never look them in the eye or be natural and relaxed. If you haven't used the honest approach, try it and see. It's like swimming: formidable in prospect, but quite natural once the unreasoning fear is gone.

Tell people they have cancer? Certainly, and at the earliest opportunity, while they're still physically strong enough to face it. And I don't think much of evasions or cute phrases like "a little tumor" or "the next thing to a cancer."

Not that I ever tell a patient his situation is hopeless. Such is the emotional armor of the human spirit that he'd refuse to believe me if I did so. "Serious," "very serious," "life threatening" are adequate for the rare man who needs to be stimulated to clean his financial house.

More important, but usually neglected, is the stimulus to have a man give power of attorney early in the course of any illness that threatens his intellect. Having him declared mentally incompetent later or having to testify as to the state of his mind when he signed important business documents can be unpleasant. I simply say, "In case it should ever be necessary, I'd suggest you give your son power of attorney to handle your affairs. That way all your bills can be paid if a time should come when you're temporarily incapacitated."

In the early stages of a terminal illness I like to take the spouse into our conferences. If doctors find it hard to discuss these matters with the dying, it's even harder for the relatives unless we break the ice first. On a few occasions I've been hogtied by strict orders from relatives not to discuss the nature of a patient's problems with him. But if the wife is there with the husband when the word is *first* given, there'll be no way for her to block me. And besides it saves time for me and puts the ring of honesty in my words to have both of them there. Most important, it prevents that horrible and futile game in which husband and wife each knows the truth but tries to keep the other from finding out. If ever a couple needs to share, it's when the going is rough. If it's important to involve the husband in the birth of his children, it's no less important to involve him in the mortal illness of his wife.

As the patient fades, others will have to take over his side of the contract. Sometimes these others will have no rapport with the doctor at all, as I learned once when I was discharged from the case of an old pensioner I'd jollied along for years. His daughter had worked for one of my competitors and, quite properly, had put her faith in him.

Generally, relatives will accept a patient's doctor if *he* does, but knowing that the outcome is probably going to be grim puts me on my mettle to pay even more attention to my relative relationships. This takes the form of getting to know them, chatting with them when our bedside visits coincide, and being cordial and helpful when they telephone me. If there's any hint that they're dissatisfied, or uncertain of my ability, I suggest a consultation right off. Usually this will reassure them that I'm confident about my handling of the case, and they'll back down. It's not that I mind a consultant at this point, but I hate to spend a patient's money and bother a colleague over a case that's clearly terminal.

Like the patient, relatives should have the longest possible preparation for the approach of death. Unlike the patient, who may be permitted to deny reality and to resort to any other protective mechanism, the relatives should be pressed a little harder to face facts. They'll *have* to face those facts in time, while he can carry his illusions into the last coma. To the extent that I leave him hope and gradually take it all away from them, I *do* work behind his back, but even that campaign can often be delayed until he's too sick to notice.

Then as we go into the last week I try to avoid the grisly death watches by cadres of funereal relatives, most of whom would far rather be bowling than bawling (and might better be) but for their fear that "the neighbors would talk" if they weren't at ringside for every terminal twitch. Others may be belatedly trying to expiate years of neglect; worst of all are the morbidly curious whose eyes dart to every tube and tumor so they'll have lurid tales to embroider at future bridge tables.

My ideal family sends one close representative at a time to sit briefly at the bedside during regular hours. Dying people shouldn't be out of human earshot, but they're in no condition to entertain near-strangers from the past. And even if my patient were able to appreciate the presence of distant relatives, their arrival would surely tell him the end was near. I've had hospital patients with a *good* prognosis shocked into near hysterics by the unexpected arrival of a son in military service, figuring he could have gotten leave only on the basis of an imminent death in the family. When flocks of moist-eyed vultures circle around *my* bed, you'd better believe I'll start checking *my* toes for flexion.

Besides, I find it much harder to console relatives who've been staying awake to the edge of exhaustion. Lack of sleep is itself depressing and we certainly don't need any augmentation of gloom at times like these.

So I say firmly: "We have some tough times just ahead. You won't be any good to your relative or to me if you're exhausted,

so I want you to go home tonight and get 10 hours of sleep—
here's a pill to make sure you rest."

Toward the end I slack off on therapy for several reasons.
When the issue is hopeless, there's no point in wasting money for
the sheer appearance of "flapping my arms." And, if death is
imminent and the patient is in pain, any measures that might
prolong life a few more hours are cruel. Herb Shriner has a
routine about the old family doctor back in Indiana that expresses it very well: "He's the kind of doctor that, if you're at death's
door, he pulls you through."

But mainly, I fold my therapeutic tent to show the relatives
that everything possible has been done and death is certain.
Because, if I were to keep shooting in antibiotics and tubes,
followed by cardiac massage, to the end, I'd only create a strong
impression that a little more tincture of heroics might have
reversed the issue.

It's necessary that close relatives see the dying patient at
intervals so they can be confronted with reality, but I don't like
them there for the agonal throes. It's horrible enough for me as
the doctor to watch those shudders and gasps. Were I to see
them in a member of my immediate family I'm afraid the sight
might blot out all the pleasant scenes we shared in life. But I'd
like to have a trusted family friend at the bedside during those
last moments, and I'm afraid no intern, resident, or nurse could
substitute for the trusted family doctor. So when it's possible, I
go and I stay. Every 15 minutes or so I come out of the room and
report to the relatives, and then I go back. It's not very productive time, and I don't charge much for it. Maybe it's my penance
for having failed—there never was a fatal case where, in retros-
pect, I haven't wished I'd done things differently.

That's an admission I often share with the relatives because
they'll have similar feelings about their own lack of prescience.

Before I leave the room for the last time, I cover the body.

Then I firmly discourage the family from going in. I wish they could be left with memories only of a living person, but at least the cruel societal rule that demands the display of dead people to the public also requires that they be painted a rosier cadaveric hue.

Instead, I shepherd the mourners into a remote and sound-proofed room—sobs and screams aren't reassuring to the convalescing, particularly if they've just been intimately exposed to the medieval system of allowing patients to rattle and groan their last in a ward bed. I give the news the relatives have already seen in my face, and then I just sit quietly.

When they're ready, I ask about funeral arrangements and then—always—offer an autopsy. Just as the offer of consultation proves my confidence, the offer of an autopsy proves I'm not trying to hide anything.

I suppose everybody comes out of internship with his own bag of tricks for getting an autopsy: My favorite tool is curiosity. Much as I'd like to convince the relatives that I know exactly what's inside, I try to leave a little doubt about some aspect of the case. ("There's a possibility that the indigestion he's complained of lately could represent an early cancer. If so, it would put an entirely new aspect on this heart attack.") Where there's genuine doubt about the primary diagnosis, I express it frankly and add, "Unless we find out for sure, you and I are going to wonder the rest of our lives whether we did everything possible." Of course, when one raises such doubts he's honor-bound to resolve them—not on the day of the autopsy, but a few weeks later when things are more comfortably remote.

Mature, intelligent relatives almost always respond to an appeal to advance medical knowledge: "It will neither hurt nor help him, but it may help us to learn more about his disease and be a little smarter about it in the future."

I suppose all these admissions of fallibility shudder malpractice insurers, and I'd certainly hate to be quoted in court. But I know that, spoken from genuine concern, my confessions close the credibility gap for good. Sometimes I'm so honest in expressing my doubts that relatives find themselves comforting me as much as I comfort them.

Which brings a poignant scene to mind: Once I was doing my best to assuage the pain of a new widow when her minister came in. She went into his arms and was held until she found comfort there, as many had before.

I knew then what the clergy have that doctors have lost to science. When I find it in myself I'll know I've achieved the ultimate in being truly a physician. It has roots in being self-confident when faced with death and grief, and in being able to do what's natural when another human being needs a pair of strong arms to fall into.

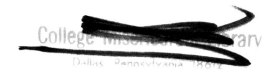